Youngevity Revolution

The 12 Secret Spirals of Enduring Youth and Longevity

Rino Soriano

Disclaimer

The material in this book is for educational purposes only, it makes no claims about your health and does not diagnose, cure or treat any condition. It is designed with the intent to make you aware of Higher faculties about your life and is mainly about lifestyle and for making healthier choices. By following the information in this book, you do so at your own choosing and agree to maintain Rino Soriano and Flying Hawk Productions and all other Affiliations harmless of any circumstances that may arise by following such information.

Table of Contents

The Youngevity Revolution – Are You Game?

Preface

Ok my friend, are you ready? Are you ready to discover the greatest health and wellness secrets to enduring youth and longevity? This book is going to rock your world! So, pay attention and begin to embody what the wisdom and knowledge in these pages presents to you. If you truly follow what is being revealed here to you, you may put yourself in a unique league of people who get to experience a healthy and long life or what I call youngevity. Youngevity is feeling fantastic, looking young, feeling young, living young and rocking this life out as your Higher Potential Self.

We as a humanity are on the cusp of something amazing. You see, with the information here in this book along with some very powerful scientific discoveries in recent years you as a human being are going to be able to extend your life by many decades and potentially indefinitely. You will also be able to maintain your health and feel absolutely fantastic for most of the days of your life. How exciting is that for you? Do you really comprehend what this means?

It means that you have the potential to live a fulfilled life and experience all the desires of your heart as you will have more time to enjoy these pleasures. Hold onto to your hat because you are in for one amazing ride. In the pages that follow, I shall reveal to you the greatest health and wellness secrets for helping you to live a life of enduring youth and longevity. These secrets are very powerful, however, you require to embody them on a daily basis if you want them to produce results that last.

Strap yourself in and prepare your mind, body and spirit for the most exciting adventure you have yet to experience. With this new knowledge you will be inspired to live your Greatest and Highest Life. Once you discover what is being presented here, you have no more excuses my friend. It shall be time for you to go out and be the Great Being that you are meant to be. No more complacency, ignorance and just sitting around. No Way!! It is time to go out and create beautiful experiences for yourself, your family and the planet. **Are you ready?**

Before you begin to learn these secret spirals of youngevity it is very important for you to clear out all the misinformation, hype, scams and erroneous beliefs about health, wellness and what you think is True. Essentially, you require detoxing your mind of the information that does not validate itself or is based on lies, illusions and misinformation. I shall begin to uncover all the erroneous myths that you have been conditioned with over the years, and there are many.

You simply can't learn new information and put it on top of the erroneous health myths. You require to clear the misinformation first and then take in new and True wisdom, knowledge and information that validates itself. You will hear me say throughout this book that there is one life philosophy that shall serve you almost every single time and that is ... **Life Will Always Reveal The Truth To You!**

I shall teach you how to discern what is True and what is simply misinformation. So, if you are ready to embark on this amazing journey of discovery and empowerment, tell yourself right now that you are willing to let go of all the misinformation and myths that you have been conditioned with.

This process may challenge you a bit because some of your greatest held beliefs about health and wellness that you think are True are going to be exposed for the misinformation they are and it may take you a little time to transition to new beliefs. Here's the deal, what I teach and reveal validates itself. This information is not my theory or something that I put together and slapped my label on it. This is a Higher level of Truth and you along with millions of people have missed this simple Truth because of all the erroneous myths and theories being sent your way almost everywhere you go. You shall begin to see life with new eyes after you are done reading this book, I assure you.

Discernment is the greatest asset you have at this point on the planet since there is way too much information now and to know what is True and what is not, well, it can be a challenge. However, that is where I come in. I shall teach you how discern and know if something is True or just another illusion, scam or myth. It is actually so simple that you miss it. It is an illusionary world out there at times so for you the greatest lesson at this time is to invest in your health and empowerment and learn discernment. Once you do then you will never be scammed again or led in a funny direction. You will be conscious and know how to navigate through the soup of life.

I am actually quite excited for you since I know this information is going to change your life dramatically and the Potential that awaits you is Grand. Happy Discovery!

Foreword

Ok my friend, I shall begin to uncover the main erroneous concepts mainly pertaining to health and wellness. Again, please prepare yourself as the information that I present may challenge your belief system. You may not even believe what I am about to share with you, however, what I present validates itself. This means you can go out and validate this in your life very simply. Usually all you will require to do is observe life with new eyes and then you shall see Truth.

Most of the health information you will find in society simply does not validate itself and does not help a majority of people. There is a main reason why…and that is because every single person has a unique biological makeup, mental makeup and spiritual composition. This means that what serves you well for health and wellness may not serve the next person or even your family members. Essentially, your health and your requirements for maintaining it are going to be unique unto you so you require learning how to tap into your inner intelligence to determine exactly what is best for you.

This is why all the health fads, diet fads and all these other health myths being proposed as the magic one way to health simply do not create health for a majority of people. You can't standardize health and say you have the holy way for everyone and put it in a package and sell it to people. That is a scam!

Your health is a combination of habits that you embody every day. These habits are unique unto you. Your body may require more or less of certain nutrients based upon your lifestyle, your body type, your occupation, your mental state and even your spiritual embodiment.

There are many paradigms out there right now. Each paradigm proclaims that they have the Holy Way to health. You name it…Vegan, Vegetarian, Raw and many others. If all of these health paradigms are so healthy and are true, then where are all the fit, healthy and radiant people? In case you do not know, is that most people these days are not healthy or radiant or fit or nowhere near that. I live by a simply philosophy and that is…**Life Shall Always Reveal The Truth To You**.

So, when I observe life and the health of people, I see most people not even coming near being healthy let alone radiant and fit. So what gives and why do the health paradigms that so many people proclaim is the holy way to health, do not produce lasting results in helping people to be fit, healthy and radiant?

The secret is that your health is a combination of holistic practices you do each day along with a state of Consciousness. Most people do not realize that your Consciousness is a vital part to your health. Without consciousness you simply cannot create optimum health let alone evolve yourself to the Highest degree. So, the way I am referring to Consciousness has to do with how you use your Consciousness on a daily basis.

Are you using it to uplift yourself and for creating your life consciously or are you using your Consciousness to actually stifle yourself as most people are doing? By using your Consciousness consciously, you allow your Highest expression of who you are. Most people are not using their Consciousness consciously, they are simply allowing their programs and unconscious behaviors to run the show.

The time has come for humanity to begin embodying a holistic process for living life. Humanity also requires becoming their own master of their life and their health. For too long humanity has been relying on external authorities and so called experts to tell them how to live and how to input nutrition into their bodies. Well, if I may be honest with you right now...that approach really hasn't done much to assist people to be healthy let alone evolve themselves. That external seeking actually pulls people from the

Truth and you end up giving your power away to someone or something else.

For thousands of years now humanity has given its power over and the results speak for themselves. I am only making observations and calling it like I see it. If you want to evolve yourself along with extending your life then you require embodying your Higher Faculties and learn to be your own master by honoring your intuition and body wisdom. That is the holy way that shall serve you and actually get you results that last.

The health paradigms being taught out there have had more than enough time to validate themselves and they simply have not. In fact, most health paradigms have done the exact opposite of what they are proclaiming. If you have the eyes to see then the Truth becomes quite apparent. Following paradigms puts you into a rigid box that does not allow you to see the Higher Truth. Following paradigms also does not get you results.

My point is each person requires determining what is best for them and you do that by going within and listening to your body wisdom and your intuition. This is the Holy Way that everyone is seeking. This is the only True way to know for sure what it is that serves your health adequately. Another important point is that you may require altering your nutrition and health habits throughout the year and throughout certain phases in your life.

Essentially, your health is fluid and changes over time so you require feeling when that is for you. Again, once you learn to tap into your inner guidance and body wisdom then you will usually know exactly what you require, when and how much. **Go Within my friend, this is the only True way to enduring health and wellness and to longevity.**

The Mysterious Demystified

A simple formula for you to follow to ensure you remain on track for optimum health is as follows: **There are only 3 factors that are the cause for health disorders and low level health.**

1) **Toxins** – these include heavy metals, viruses, parasites

2) **Nutrient Deficiencies** – these include water, vitamins, minerals, trace elements, essential fatty acids, amino acids, anti-oxidants, sunlight

3) **Emotional, mental and spiritual deficiencies** – resolving these can dramatically improve your health and well-being.

The time has come where each human being take responsibility for their whole lives. Your health is the greatest asset you have. With optimal health you can then go out and experience this life with a Higher Consciousness and a great feeling. You will also be inspired to do great things as your feeling of health and wellness shall cause your Higher faculties to kick in and serve as fuel for your spiritual evolution.

It is quite amazing to see when someone is radiantly health. You can see it in their eyes and feel it in their vibration. They simply are fun to be around and get stuff done. They are creative and always looking to help people, animals and planet. These are quite extraordinary people and when you meet one of them you absolutely know as they have something remarkable about them. Well, you can be one of these people my friend. You have the potential. The question…are you willing to do what it takes to be one?

The Greatest Secret Of The Universe

Ok, so I think you are beginning to see that just because you believe something to be True does not necessarily mean that it is True. Humanity has created many belief systems and paradigms in the past few thousand years and it has actually caused many people to become stifled in their evolution. I am here to present to you Higher Truth and wisdom that validates itself with results that you can see and feel. So, if you will allow yourself to be open minded, you shall see that what I teach is a Higher way of living this life which in turn shall assist you on your evolutionary journey.

So, what I am about to share with you is only know by a few enlightened beings at this time and has only been known by a few others to walk this planet in the past few thousand or more years. You are very blessed to discover this wisdom as this can serve to catapult your evolution and place you on path to actually extending your life by many years and more.

There are many scientists and researchers that have for many years attempted to discover the fountain of youth. They have pondered and experimented and have created many theories of how they believe they can extend human life. On one level it is a good thing to want to discover how to extend human life and create a healthier life as well. However, the way these scientists are going at attempting to discover the secret to longevity is not the direction that shall help them to actually discover anything of substance.

You see, scientists are using an erroneous process for looking at life based on conventional scientific models that obviously haven't produced any significant advancements. Also, the perspective that scientists are using is not going to allow them to see the Higher Truth that is starring right at them every day. For thousands of years now, humans have been looking at life as a physical creation with physical substances and physical bodies, whether stars, planets and even a human body. They view the Universe as a physical creation with physical molecules that make up physical stuff. And there lies the quandry!!!

The secret is that there are no physical particles in the Universe, never have been and never will. Your body is also not made up of physical molecules and other physical substances. This Higher level of Truth is why most scientists have not been able to make any viable sense of this Universe and life on planet earth. They keep hitting cosmic walls because they are viewing the Universe as a physical thing which it clearly is not.

Albert Einstein stated: *"Concerning matter, we have been all wrong. What we have called matter is energy, whose vibration has been so lowered as to be perceptible to the senses. There is no matter."* All matter beings vibrate at specific rates and everything has its own melody.

The musical nature of matter and atoms is now finally being recognized by science. (Excerpt From AttunedVibration.com)

So, if the Universe is not physical then what is it? Ah ha...there lies the secret. Are you ready to discover the greatest secret to ever be presented to humanity? Are you ready to have your paradigms rocked outside the galaxy? Ok, here it is...There are only 2 things that exist in this Universe, one is called Consciousness and the other is called photons or what some call Light.

This grand Universe is a grand Light Show and the thing powering it is called Consciousness. Ding Dong, hello, are you there? Do you understand what this means? Do you comprehend the profundity of this discovery? I pray you do because if you get it, and I mean truly get it, you will soon discover the secret to evolution and extending your life by many decades and perhaps longer.

Your body is not made up of physical molecules as scientists say it is. It is made up of condensed Light. At the Essence level your cells and DNA are vibrating Light photons.

Quantum science is just beginning to tap into this Higher Truth. And because your body is really made up of condensed Light, you can do things to easily alter and change the Light Photons with your Consciousness. What this means is you can alter and program your body to be healthy and to live a super long life when you get in tune with your True Essence. When you learn how to honor and nurture and nourish your body as a Sacred Temple, then you shall begin to see miracles in your health and life. When you learn how to use your Consciousness consciously and choose to create a healthy and vibrant body, you will see and feel things that will leave you marveling. Do you get this?

This means you can direct and change the Light photons to be what you want them to be using your Consciousness and Awareness. This is how the entire Universe functions by the way. Consciousness directs the photons to be what they are.

"The forms of snowflakes and faces of flowers may take on their shape because they are responding to some sound in nature. Likewise, it is possible that crystals, plants, and human beings may be, in some way, music that has taken on visible form."

Quote by Hans Jenny

How do you think your body is functioning right now? What do you think is powering your body and directing the billions of biological processes that happen in even just one second? My friend, it is Consciousness doing it. Even if you put together thousands of the most advanced computers on the planet they would not be able to do what the human body does, not even for one second. Talk about amazing and mysterious.

So, if you want to extend your life then you are going to require purging all of the erroneous philosophies and programs that you have accepted as Truth. What I have just revealed is literally humanity's bridge to quantum evolution. It is revolutionary in the aspect that you are the creator of your life and your body. So, if you want to change your life and your body then use your Consciousness consciously. Yes, it is this simple. Your belief systems and programs aren't going to want to hear this right now as it means they are done and shall have no more life. However, until you pur-ge these programs and belief systems, they will stifle your evolution.

I have just revealed the most profound secret to life that you will ever discover. With this discovery, you are now at the steering wheel of your health and your life. No more excuses and no more seeking. You are the Consciousness that directs the Light Photons to create what you intend. I call this conscious creation and is the way humanity is supposed to live life. This is why most philosophies and paradigms are pulling most people away from the Truth. Most paradigms are programming you with misin-formation. When you learn to rely on your intuition and body wisdom then you no longer can be programmed or manipulated. You shall just know Truth from within.

When humanity begins to view life and their body as Light, this is when you will see quantum shifts in evolution and the restructuring of human life on this planet. For too long, humanity has been hoodwinked into placing their Consciousness externally and distractions of philosophies and other erroneous paradigms. In doing so, they have given their creation powers away and have caused themselves to be stifled.

Are you ready to accept the Truth that you are part of the Conscious-ness that created the Universe? Are you willing to step into your Great-ness and begin using your Consciousness consciously for the Greater Good Of All? It is only in this way that we are going to change this Sacred Planet and live fruitful lives. Take your power back right now and use your Consciousness to create a thrilling life journey. It is your creation so why not create an extraordinary story for yourself and planet Earth.

The Proof Has Been There For Quite Some Time

A few years ago, scientists were baffled at some experiments they were performing across the planet. They were doing the same experiment at various geographic regions around the planet using the same controls and variables. What they were experiencing was that each of the re-searchers from different countries were all coming up with different and unique outcomes of the same experiment. They were quite baffled for a bit of time and so they continued to run the experiment and kept coming up with different outcomes from each of the researchers who performed the experiment. They kept pondering of how was this so if they all used the same controls and all used the same input variables into the experiment, how were there different outcomes among all of the researchers? The answer was quite simple as they found out. It was the Consciousness of each researcher that was affecting the outcome of the experiment. It was found out after many runs of the experiment that each researcher's beliefs and biased opinions of what they thought was going to be the outcome actually caused the outcome to match very closely to what they believed they would see.

Do you see what this validates now? **This proves that your Consciousness can and does alter reality.** My friend, you are the creator of your entire life. Your ego does not want to hear this because it means that you are responsible for your entire life. Most people simply do not want to come to this realization because it means they have to be sharp and authentic and extraordinary and they have to drop their story of who they think they are. Your ego wants you to play small and not know that you are the Creator of your life. As long as you do not know this fact then you can play complacent and small and live a comfortable life like most people choose to do unconsciously. I am not here to judge, I am stating a fact that has been so for thousands of years.

The Universe is not the one drilling you over and over again and your past does not determine who you are today although it does for most people because they choose to believe it is so and therefore they get to be right. It is time to wake up and step into who you truly are. The Universe is a mirror and delivers to you what you believe to be True. So, if you do not like your life then I must inform you that you are the only one creating it and you have the power to change it. Praying to a God in the heavens is giving your power over and that really has not been too effective over thousands of years for most of humanity.

Perhaps you may begin praying inward to yourself, to your heart and then maybe, just maybe you will begin to see the miracles you have been waiting for. After all, you are the Consciousness that directs the Light photons to arrange in specific shapes and sizes. Yes, my friend, this is of Truth. You can disbelieve all you want, however, until you come to this direct realization of who you truly are then you will continue to create limitations for yourself and perpetuate the disharmony of planet Earth.

Consciousness is the key to life, to the Universe and to your health. **Consciousness powers everything and is your link to Source and the gateway to your expansion and evolution.** With Consciousness you can create anything you want because it directs the Light photons. It is now your choice of what you do with this profound wisdom. Choose wisely!

May The Force Be With You

What I am about to reveal shall catapult your Consciousness to Higher grounds. You see, this expansive Universe is a sea of many frequencies. Everything in the entire Universe has its own unique frequency signature. In essence, everything is blipping out a frequency, a song if you will. Every being on this planet is singing a song that ripples out. At the fundamental level, everything has what is called Life Force.

In the aspect of your body and health, you have Life Force permeating each one of your cells, otherwise, you simply would not be able to function let alone live. Life Force is the foundation to who you are and is the Essence to your True Being. Life Force is the most valuable asset you have in your life. With Life Force, you can do and create extraordinary things in life. Life Force is the powerhouse that creates magic. You require Life Force to evolve and to have a healthy body. In fact, having an abundance of Life Force is the key to extending your life by many decades and beyond.

Some of the Asian cultures and some other indigenous cultures have known about the significance of Life Force and thus is the reason why they structure their lives ensuring they keep an abundance of it. Life Force is your link to Higher States of Consciousness and for being able to tap into your Higher Potentials. It is your pathway to True Evolution.

However, most people do not know of this fact. Most people are depleting their Life Force on a daily basis and as such you get what you got on this planet. A majority of humanity is depleted of Life Force and thus you have a society that is not in tune with their True Self. Simply look and observe and there you have the byproducts of when humans have very little Life Force in their lives.

You deplete your Life Force every time you engage in any activity that is lowering your frequency or taking energy away from you. In this modern society, there are many, many activities that are doing so for most people. Activities such as drinking unstructured water, consuming nutrient devoid foods, consuming unhealthy food and drink products, smoking, drinking alcohol, listening to disharmonic music, getting angry at someone, having sex which has no love involved, going to a job that you do not enjoy, being with partner you are not in love with, not getting grounded with Mother

Earth on a regular basis, and the list goes on. Most people are doing activities every day that are depleting their Life Force.

Most of society is set up in a way that is depleting to you and your Life Force. I call it the Hamster Wheel where you are going and going and you really are not going anywhere and you are depleting your Life Force. Until humanity wakes up from this toxic cycle of spinning their wheels with no results in evolution, they will continue to deplete their Life Force. Once your Life Force is used up, guess what…Lights out.

Once the body runs out of Life Force, you can no longer live and this is the reason why most people live short lives. They have run out of Life Force because they depleted it by living a life not on purpose, living in a toxic manner, ingesting food that has no Life Force in it, drinking water that has no Life Force in it, having superficial sex, going to a job that provided no joy or happiness, lived with a partner that was not in Alignment with their Truth, drank alcohol on a regular basis, smoked and did many other activities that are Life Force depletors.

I am simply shedding Light on the Truth. Society living is toxic to human health and evolution. It is not supposed to be this way my friend. So, if you are wanting to extend your life and be healthy, then you are going to require embodying a Holistic Process and change many things about your life and the way you live your life, otherwise, you will most likely have the same results as most people. Life Force is the Secret Key to evolution and your life of health and longevity.

"Life Force is the Light. Life Force is your Light. Life Force is your power of creation. Life Force is the elixir of life. Life Force illuminates your Consciousness. Life Force is the magic essence of your soul. Life Force is the pathway to your Higher Potentials. Life Force is the pathway to Longevity and beyond."

Rino Soriano

The 5 Pillars of Evolution and Longevity

There are 5 key pillars of evolution or what I call Life Force Generators that are the pathway to your evolution and longevity. If you truly desire to evolve yourself and live an extended life then embodying these Life Force Generators will be essential on your evolutionary journey. These 5 key pillars shall provide the foundation for your expansion and they will continue to generate Life Force for you as to be your power supply of energy, inspiration and love.

1) Optimum Health – your evolution is dependent upon how healthy your body is and how free flowing your Life Force is running through your energy meridians. Life Force flows through your body via energy meridians and as long as it flows freely, your body tends to be healthy and vibrant. Your body is a Sacred Temple and when you treat it as such you get to experience life on a much Higher level. Your body is not a machine as most people think it is where they just dump anything in without regards to what it is doing to their Sacred System.

Your body is a living Sacred Temple that houses the Conscious Life Force. Do you understand what I am saying right now? Ok, so I shall put it another way just to make sure you get it. Your body is a Sacred Temple because it houses the Consciousness that created the Universe. The Consciousness, Infinite Spirit, Creator Source, The Light that created the Universe permeates every single cell in your body and instructs each cell to do what it does. Only Consciousness can power the billions of biochemical processes that happen in your body every second.

Only Consciousness can keep an organization of every single cellular process and do it perfectly day in and day out. No machine or computer ever can do what Consciousness does. Do you got it now? I pray you do because until you embody this Truth you will probably continue to treat your body like a machine which then simply won't allow you to extend your life let alone evolve yourself to the Highest degree. The implications are quantum my friend. Your body is the pathway to your evolution so thus you require learning how to care for it and treat it as a Sacred Temple, because it is.

2) Living Your Passion – One of the greatest feelings in life is when you are Aligned with your True Self and living your passion. Living your passion is essentially being involved in any activity or process that gives you great inspiration and feeds your spirit. You can easily see and feel when someone is living their passion. There is a glow about them, an energy they carry that simply affects everyone and everything around them. Being in tune with yourself and living your Truth is to be in Alignment with your Soul. Being in this frequency literally elevates your Consciousness and also your body. Your body produces many life enhancing bio-chemicals when you are in a state of bliss and happiness. Living your passion generates lots of love and joy in your heart and thus your body then produces bio-chemicals that uplift your health and also your level of Consciousness.

There is a secret that your body houses. Your body has an immaculate endocrine system and hormone system. Essentially your body is a

Divine factory of many life enhancing bio-chemicals that can uplift your being and regenerate your body. The fountain of youth is housed within your endocrine and hormone systems. And here is the most profound secret to longevity... **it is your state of being that determines what kind of bio-chemicals get produced by your body.**

If you are unhappy and stressed out then your body will produce bio-chemicals that mirror this internal consciousness state and thus sets you up for degeneration and low level health. If you are in a state of bliss, joy, love and happiness then your body easily produces life enhancing bio-chemicals that regenerate and rejuvenate your body system. The implications are multi-dimensional as these life enhancing bio-chemicals also will elevate your mood and serve to be a catalyst for emotional and mental well-being, clarity, calm and an overall sense of connection to life.

The next time you are happy and blissed out simply notice how you feel in your body and notice how you feel not only physically well but also mentally and emotionally well. This is a direct reflection of your body producing life enhancing bio-chemicals that impact your body and brain and ripple out to your entire state of being. My friend, your body already houses the fountain of youth. It is a Universal Truth! The question is... are you going to allow this Truth to be embodied in your life? Only you can structure your life and use your Consciousness as to experience this Truth for yourself.

So, as you can see, living your passion is absolutely essential for your evolution and expansion as a being. It is one of the most profound experiences in life. So, if you value yourself and your life, then do everything you can to discover what your passions are and then go out and live them.

Maybe it is playing music, or maybe doing art, or it can even be a career that you find so thrilling to be in. Whatever it is only you know because you will feel it in your body when you are living your passion. This energy that gets generated by living your passion literally keeps your cells and body healthy and young. It is the juice that catapults your full being to Higher Possibilities. This planet could easily be transformed if more people were honoring and living their passion. Most people settle and live lives that they really do not want to by trying to fit in, trying to bo cuoocooful, trying to impress, trying to be right and a whole list of other life depleting life activities that do not feed their Soul.

If you truly desire to expand yourself then you require being honest with yourself. This means you sit with yourself and go deep within and discover what is it that brings your heart bliss and passion? What inspires you and what energizes you? Only you know and only you can make the decision to honor and follow and live your passion. So, what are you waiting for? Just so you know, the entire Universe gives you permission to go for it, to live your passion and Light your life up. The only one holding you back is YOU. Go live your passion because it is the most essential path for your evolution. You owe to it humanity to live your passion because you allow your Higher Potentials to come forth. You also serve to be a model for others and give them permission to go live their passions. This is bigger than you my friend, living your passion has global implications that can affect many people. Now go out there and **LIVE YOUR PASSION!!!**

3) Alignment With Your Soul – To be Aligned with your Soul is to be in direct knowing of your True Self. What this means is you know who you truly are deep down inside. To be Aligned and in tune with your Soul is the greatest connection to have in life. It serves as your navigation system for traversing this soup of life. Your Soul is your connection to Source and All That Is. It is your fulcrum and foundation to experience life on a multi-dimensional level.

Being Aligned with your Soul allows you to experience life with new eyes and inspirational feelings of love and honor for all life on planet Earth. It is the way we are all supposed to be living. When people are Aligned with their Soul they naturally want to live clean lives and be kind to others. They naturally care for the planet and live simply as they know that the way we treat the planet has a direct effect on us. Aligned people are gentle and loving and have a deep sense of care for all of humanity and the planet.

This modern society has gotten way off path from Truth. Simply look and there you have people who are not in Alignment with Soul. They are functioning out of belief systems and superficial processes for living life. As such, many people are not in Alignment with their Soul so thus they do not see and feel spiritual things nor care to the degree they could. Most of humanity is not Aligned with Soul and as such you have what you got on this planet. I call it being unconscious and unaligned.

Only an unconscious humanity would allow the planet to be stripped and trashed in order to satisfy ego desires and wants. Only unconscious beings would allow an entire eco planetary system to be converted into one big shopping mall where everything and anything is for sale.

Aligning with your Soul is really the only True Substance that you will ever require to live an amazing life. Your Soul will reveal so many uplifting Truths to you when you are ready. Your Soul shall guide you throughout your life and be your inspiration for living life with passion and bliss. Soul Alignment is the fulcrum to your evolution. It is the only way that you shall ever feel satisfied with anything in life. Soul is the Universal Substance that shall catapult you to the stars. **Align with your Soul and see miracles opening up in your life.** Soul is the Way my friend!

4) Connection With Others of Like Mind

Connecting with others of like mind is an essential ingredient for your expansion. You see, being with others who share similar lifestyles and philosophies of life is a great Life Force Generator. When two or more people come together for a common purpose, there is a vast amount of energy generated. In this energy and space, there are many potentials and miracles possible. It seems that everyone who comes into this field of energy or Life Force gets catapulted in Consciousness and in well-being.

Feeling the love and support of others of like mind on your spiritual journey is one of the greatest resources of inspiration. Your connection with others can significantly help you to manifest a higher reality for yourself with the positive energies and the support you feel you have in the field of connection. Look at this way... if you had to elevate a BIG stone that weighed 100 pounds, do you think you can do this easier by yourself or with two other people giving you support? The feeling of being supported and assisted by others can dramatically elevate your confidence in going through life with a Higher perspective and a Higher knowing that you can do almost anything you put your mind to.

The connection with others of like mind creates a synergy that everyone in the field of that space can feel it and gets inspired to go out in life and rock. It keeps everyone in that space motivated to do greater things, to be nicer, to be more authentic and to simply be all in for the greater good of all.

Perhaps you can begin going out and connecting with more people of like mind. Search online as there are many groups forming on various topics of life. You will easily discover groups of people of like mind that you can go connect with on a regular basis. You may require to step outside of your comfort zone a bit. It is ok, do it anyway. The time is at hand and it benefits you to begin expanding your boundaries and having new experiences.

Also, you shall notice that your health improves when you are in connection with others of like mind. This is because your body and brain are producing bio-chemicals that uplift your health. It has been shown scientifically that when people connect at the heart level and love is present, the people in that space are being uplifted in health and wellness. Love is the greatest elixir of life and can create miracles. So, perhaps you can begin your expansion journey to allowing more love and connection in your life. You will be amazed at the results. Happy Connecting!!!

5) Consciousness

Consciousness is the most important component to your life. It is your Consciousness that is the absolute foundation to what you experience in life and how high you can evolve yourself. Mainly, it is how you are using your Consciousness that determines what the Universe reflects back to you with life experiences. The Universe is your mirror and is always reflecting to you what you are creating with your Consciousness. However, most people are creating unconsciously in their life. They are using outdated belief systems to attempt to create their life which is constantly changing and shifting.

Outdated belief systems are the greatest hindrances to expansion and evolution. Humanity for thousands of years now has been attempting to use belief systems and paradigms to create in life. Well, if I may be honest for even just one second with you, that process for creating life has not been too good for humanities' expansion let alone being healthy for this planet. If you simply observe the Truth shall become quite apparent that belief systems have stifled humanity now for thousands of years. Belief systems create separation and limitations. Belief systems do not allow expansion let alone the possibility for harmony.

Belief systems put you inside a box and keep you rigid in your philosophies. This rigidness literally keeps you perpetuating the same patterns over and over again. It is like watching the same tv show over and over again day after day. How can you or anyone for that matter even begin to expand themselves or evolve with this rigidness? It is not possible.

If we as a humanity are going to create Higher Potentials for ourselves and for future generations, then we require to shed belief systems altogether. We require living on Universal Truths. Universal Truths are self-validating and allow for expansion. Universal Truths supply a foundation on which you can then use for creating Higher Potentials. For example, the Universal Truth that the sun rises in the east and sets in the west is easily observable and has been so for millions of years. You do not require believing this to be so for it to be a Truth. It just is. There are many Universal Truths that we can use to serve as a foundation for our expansion. We simply require using a Higher Consciousness.

In my teachings I call it using Luminous Consciousness. **Luminous Consciousness is like using a brilliant light to shine on any topic of life and using the Highest Universal Truths as to consciously create a life experience that benefits as many people as possible.**

Luminous Consciousness illuminates a Higher Consciousness perspective as to allow for expansion and evolution. There are no belief systems in Luminous Consciousness because you function on Universal Truths that are self-validating and serve to uplift all of life. There is also a Higher Connection to Intuition and other Higher Faculties when you are in Luminous Consciousness. Some may call it embodying a Christ Consciousness where you use your heart and soul to guide you and to intuit Higher Universal Truths that come from Spirit/Source.

Luminous Consciousness is the pathway for humanities' expansion and True evolution. It is the bridge into a Higher Reality that is based on service to others and love. You can begin embodying this level of

Consciousness for yourself starting immediately. How you may ask? Well, you can begin by becoming more conscious of your internal feelings and seeking to connect with that aspect of yourself that is in Alignment with your Higher Self. You may call upon this aspect of yourself to come forth and assist you in your expansion. You can ask for seeing a Higher Perspective of yourself and your place in this Universe. You can ask for guidance and direction as to how best to begin this conscious expansion journey.

Consciousness & Light

As I stated earlier, there really is only one thing that exists and that is Light or what some call photons. This Light or Consciousness puts forth conscious thought and thus creates matter and energy. So, matter and energy is really an expansion of the Consciousness of the Universe. The matter that you see is really only a Light show springing forth as a cosmic movie being created in the Mind of the One Consciousness that pervades this Universe and beyond. So matter gets created by Consciousness via information and energy.

Picture it like this, the One Consciousness has conscious thought that generates energy and gets things flowing and thus ripples out to then create matter. Matter is simply energy slowed down to a very perceivable level, however, it is only energy and not the solid stuff you think you see. Everything in the Universe is oscillating energy and Light. It will always be a mystery as to how this is being done on a cosmic level. It is quite beautiful when you see if from a place of simply observing and appreciating it for the glorious Light show that it is.

Using Your Consciousness Consciously

Your Consciousness is like a garden with very rich soil. Your Consciousness will sprout forth any seeds you place into it in the form of beliefs, thoughts and feelings about any topic of life. Most people are using their Consciousness unconsciously and allowing their outdated belief systems, opinions and feelings to plant seeds that then sprout forth unwanted experiences. Most people get imprinted with limiting belief systems from their family and society as children and thus this sets them up for planting seeds in their Consciousness that then attracts experiences into their life that they really do not consciously want.

It will be in your best interest to look at your belief systems and your programming from childhood and begin to clear out all outdated opinions and feelings that you have that are unhealthy or limiting in any way. Every opinion you have about any topic of life is essentially a belief system and can set you up for limitations. Perhaps you may begin simply noticing your beliefs as they come up when you are in conversation with someone. You will be amazed at how many beliefs you are carrying. You may also listen to others as they speak and notice how many beliefs they are speaking out. You come to discover that most of what people are saying are belief systems of what they think it True.

Your Consciousness will reflect back to you what your beliefs are through the Universe via life experiences. It shall boggle your mind how perfect this process is. Every minor detail of your life experiences is a reflection of what seeds you have in your Consciousness. Perhaps you will begin planting new seeds from now on?

In the aspect of longevity, you can begin using this plating new seeds principle as to set a foundation for creating a healthier and younger body. Again, matter follows the energy via your Consciousness. So, if in your Consciousness you have thoughts and feelings of looking young and living a super long life then this generates energy and begins flowing through your body which then allows for you to feel and look better. Your Consciousness is the garden with rich soil, so if you want to experience longevity then plant seeds of youthfulness and health and vitality and beauty.

Belief Systems & Paradigms: The Impediments To Evolution

I want to share with you a new perspective about beliefs and being in a paradigm. You see, beliefs are one of the greatest impediments to your evolution. How is this so you may ask? Well, in essence beliefs can serve to stifle you and place limits on what you can experience. For example, if you believe you can do only 20 push-ups in 1 minute then you are actually placing a limit on your abilities to get stuff done. What if you can do 35 to 40 push-ups in a minute if you simply use a Higher Consciousness level about yourself and your ability to perform?

You see, most people limit themselves with their beliefs and as such they get to be right since they are the Creators of their lives and the Universe is always listening and assisting you in your creations. The Universe has no biased feelings about what you create, it just puts forth in motion the energies to actually deliver to you what you are choosing to create with your beliefs and feelings.

If you look at the current state of the planet you will see what belief systems have done to people and the planet. Simply go around the planet and observe the disharmony and chaos of the byproducts of humanity's belief systems. Belief systems are the greatest impediment to evolution as they literally act like a parking brake on a car that simply does not allow you go forward. If you have your parking brake on in your car, how you can drive anywhere?

Humanity has had parking brakes on their spiritual expansion now for thousands of years because they have allowed themselves to be inebriated with erroneous belief systems. Simply look at life and there you can see plenty of examples of how humans love to have belief systems. People love feeling they are right over others. They love feeling like they are part of a group that has it right over others. Well, this level of consciousness is very limiting and simply look at the planet and see what humans have done and are doing to themselves because they feel they are right.

Just so you know is that most paradigms and belief systems have been created by people who think they have the Truth. Thinking you have the Truth and actually knowing the Truth are 2 different things. **Truth comes from Source…The Universe and nature always reveals that Truth when you have the eyes to see.** Humans have created belief systems and paradigms and the results speak for themselves. Beliefs and paradigms stifle human evolution because they are not based on Universal principles, they are based on ego perspectives that have very little substance.

If humanity is going to do anything productive and evolve themselves then the time has come to surrender beliefs systems and begin embodying Universal Truths as these are the foundation on which humans can create consciously. Universal Truths validate themselves with results that you can see and feel.

Part 2

Demystifying The Common Health Myths

Are you ready to discover the greatest health myths ever presented to you? Again, prepare yourself to shed these illusions as they are hindering your ability to create an optimal level of health. In fact, some of these erroneous myths have done more to keep you and other people unwell than to benefit your health. Here we go my friend, the most common health philosophies are about to be exposed.

The Low Fat Myth

You probably may believe that it is healthy to eat a low fat diet and to limit your total fat intake each day, correct? Well, this is actually one of the greatest scams ever created. Many people have done a disservice to their health and their families by following this erroneous philosophy. Let me present some basic science facts for you so that you may learn to discern the Truth of this topic as it is crucial for you to know.

Regardless of what has been presented to you on this topic, the simple science fact is...**fat is the most essential nutrient your body requires for optimal health**. It is required for many biological processes in your body and is a precursor to hormone production.

What this means is that your body requires a consistent supply of the right kinds of fat in order for you to have the right hormone levels in your body, along with keeping your immune system strong and for skin, hair, eyes and brain health. If you reduce total fat from your diet, you are going to alter your hormone chemistry along with being deficient in essential fatty acids that are required for optimum biological processes.

Thus you may experience improper health and functioning of your body. **Also, fats are the greatest source of energy.** Do you comprehend what this means? It means that you will actually have greater energy levels if you consume healthy fats on a consistent basis.

So, by consuming healthy levels of fat every day, you are easily increasing your energy levels. The myth that says fat makes you fat is actually false and has been proven scientifically. The Truth is by consuming healthy fats on a consistent basis you will actually moderate and improve your metabolism. This means that you will actually lose weight or maintain a healthy weight level. Fat does not make you fat. Ingesting fat does not ever get converted into fat that your body stores in various places like you have been led to believe. That is so erroneous and cannot be proven scientifically.

Everything you ingest gets broken down into smaller components on a molecular level. For example, if you ingest protein... the body transforms it into base molecules called amino acids. In the aspect of ingesting fat, your body will also break this down into smaller core molecules called lipids or simple fat compounds that your body requires for health. Actually fat gets broken down into 2 core components after you ingest it. The one is water and the other is lipids which your body takes in both as nutrition, plain and simple science.

You can validate this simple Truth by embodying this information in your daily nutrition intake. Keep in mind that you require to ingest the right kinds of fats, not just any type. What has been discovered around the world is that the cultures that ingest moderate to high amounts of healthy fats are the healthiest people on the planet. There are 2 main types of fat your body requires to be optimally healthy. One is called unsaturated fats that come from primarily plant and seeds. The other type of fat your body requires for health is called saturated fat.

In fact, saturated fat is the most essential fat your body requires for health since it is a precursor to hormone production. Without enough of this type of fat in your nutrition intake, your body cannot produce the base molecules to create hormones. Also, your metabolism cannot be at optimal levels since your metabolism is governed by hormones. In fact, every major biological process in your body is governed by hormones.

Saturated fat comes primarily from animal fats and is your KING of fats. Humans are considered animals scientifically speaking, therefore, humans must ingest animal fats to be healthy. Again, this is simple science and validates itself. The molecular structure of animal fats is the ideal form for humans to be healthy due to the fact of it being a requirement for hormone production. Your body can not produce hormones using plant or seed fats.

The molecular structure is not in the form for your body to use as the base for hormones. The common health paradigms are teaching you to stay away from saturated fats saying that they are unhealthy. Well my friend, that is not true and there is more than enough scientific data to validate that saturated fats help humans to be super healthy and strong.

Simply research the discoveries of Weston A. Price and the Truth shall be granted to you. Also, if you simply use life as your validator then that is all you require to see and feel the Truth of anything. Life will validate the Truth to you.

Every culture to ever walk the planet has ingested animal fat and protein. In fact, the healthiest cultures ever are the ones to ingest moderate to high amounts of saturated fats. The Eskimos are by far the healthiest group of people to ever walk the planet. They ingest super high amounts of fatty animal protein and other fatty compounds like raw animal milk and whale blubber and virtually no sugars or starch foods and yet they have thriving health and wellness. This is simple science my friend.

The funny theories out there presenting to you so called healthy nutrition intake are way off and counter health. Follow nature and you will fare very good. Follow theories and myths and you get what you got on this planet with most people not doing well in health especially in the USA.

The fats that are harming people are the altered and hydrogenated forms. These fats are quite toxic to the system and these are the oils that are causing improper health in many people. Hydrogenated oils are super high heated and altered from their natural composition. When you heat a compound, you alter it on a molecular level and thus create something new. In the aspect of oils, when they are heated they are changed and become toxic to your system. These oils are the ones to stay away from.

Thus, oils like margarine, Crisco, vegetable oils, canola oil, corn oil, soy oil, Wesson oil, and the whole list of altered oils are the ones to stay away from regardless of what you may think. Canola oil has been presented as a healthy oil. Well, if you do some research it has been discovered to be toxic over long term use. If you learn about where it comes from and how it is processed then the Truth is that it is not a healthy oil to consume.

The Healthiest Fats

The healthy fats are natural, unaltered and very healthy for your body. **These fats include avocado, olive oil, grapeseed oil, coconut oil, walnut oil, almond oil, macadamia nut and palm oil and butter.** Be aware that it is not healthy to cook with most oils from the fact that you alter the composition when you heat the oil.

So, my recommendation is to use steam, roasting, and grilling with a little water to cook your meals and then at the completion when your food is fully cooked after you take it off the heat, then add your oil. So, for example, if you make a soup, place all the ingredients into the pot with water and then cook it until the soup is done. Now add your oil and spices to flavor and add the healthy component of the fat. If you do require to use oil to cook with, I recommend to use coconut oil and grapeseed oil as these have high smoking points and can be used safely if you cook with them quickly. **Myth #1 exposed and vaporized!**

The Cardiovascular Myth

Here is another myth that has been presented as Truth, however, does not validate itself. **Engaging in cardiovascular endurance activities at high levels several times per week is not conducive to optimum health.** You know the activities I am talking about…aerobics, running, marathons, treadmill, and other activities and sports that result is extended elevation of heart levels. Let me clarify.

Your body is equipped with some Divine capabilities and with reserve systems that help it to function and repair. The main point here is that if you engage in high intensity cardiovascular activities on a routine basis, you are actually depleting your body and your reserves to adequately repair and regenerate.

The current health paradigm is teaching you to go out 3 to 5 days a week at 45 minutes to 1 hour to do cardio activities. It is recommended to go at 60 to 75% of maximum heart rate capability. This is ludicrous to say the least. Where this came from I have no idea but let me give you a good example of what this philosophy is saying. Essentially, it is like running your car at 75% of its maximum capability on a consistent basis. It is like stomping on the gas pedal at a stop light to go every time.

Or, another example is if you have a manual stick shift car, it is like driving your car using first and second gear only with revving the engine on a daily basis at high RPM levels. Do you think you car's engine will last long by running it in this manner? In fact, by doing this, the engine will burn out much faster.

Well, this is what people are doing to themselves by engaging in high intensity and long duration cardiovascular activities. Essentially, they are elevating their heart levels too high and potentially causing themselves harm over the long term. In fact, if you want to shorten your life span then this is one way to do that. So, the main point is, it is not healthy to engage in high intensity long duration activities and also unnecessary.

Your heart doesn't require this type of stimulation to be healthy. Yes, you require being active, you just need to do it in a healthy manner. In fact, it is best to keep your heart rate at low to moderate levels when engaging in sport activities. This is why lifting weights in the right manner or hiking with a backpack on with weight is the greatest activity you can do for looking and feeling your best. By lifting weights properly and for the right duration, you do so many awesome things for your health.

First, your body will produce many life regenerating hormones that will keep you young looking and feeling young. Second, you will put on muscle mass which in turn will help to keep your weight healthy by moderating your metabolism and you get the benefit of looking awesome. How amazing that a simple activity like lifting weights or hiking can do so many awesome things for your health. This is the #1 activity to engage in if you want to add many years to your life.

There are also other processes going on with working out with weights as in strengthening your ligaments and tendons and also mental and emotional components that most people have no clue that comes from lifting weights. Again, you require to lift weights in the right manner otherwise, you are wasting time, money and energy. I can show anyone how to do it in the right manner. It is actually so simple yet most people are unaware.

What they teach at the gym, well, this is not very effective for most people because it is over working your muscles and then the nutrition habits of most people does not support maximum gains in health and building muscle. I will now give you a simple example that shall help you to see the Truth of how high endurance long duration activities are not healthy. If you simply observe the difference between a marathon runner and a sprinter the Truth becomes quite apparent. Whom do you think is healthier and has a better functioning body?

The Truth is that the sprinter is way healthier than the marathon runner. In fact, not even close. The marathon runner is depleted and week compared to the sprinter. The marathon runner's activity and lifestyle don't allow for the body to recuperate or regenerate so thus they are in a catabolic (weak, degenerating) state.

In essence, their training and their activity is too depleting on the body and is never allowed to recuperate properly, thus simply looking at them will tell the tale and the Truth of the matter. The sprinter on the other hand is in anabolic phase and as is quite evident by simply observing their body, they are quite healthy looking and feeling. These athletes have high power, strength and musculature.

Their body is in anabolic phase meaning they are regenerating and building muscle on a routine basis. Their activity is short duration and so is their training. This is the key and one of the main secrets for engaging in fitness activities.

You see, the body absolutely requires to be worked out, however, you require to do it in the right manner otherwise it has the opposite effect.

Your muscles and body have only so many available nutrients, hydration and ATP energy to perform in activities. The intention is to engage in activities where you are using readily available bio-nutrients that your body has to give.

You want to avoid engaging in either long duration sports or activities or high intensity activities that cause you to dip into your reserve supply of energy and nutrients. This is why most athletes have short careers because they consistently place their body into tapping into reserves and they never allow their body to recuperate adequately.

The main key is to engage in activities that are short duration or start stop sports. Sports like tennis, volleyball, lifting weights, pilates, hiking, power walking and other similar short duration or start stop activities are ideal for optimal health. These activities do not cause your body to dip into reserves as much as other sports. The other main key is to fully allow the body to recuperate after engaging in your activity.

The secret is you can actually get in better shape by let's say working out with weights for only 25 to 30 minutes than if you spend 1 hour or more as most people do. In fact, the results are quite amazing when you see someone who does the proper weight training program as I teach, and the results they get with actually doing less.

So, my main point to you is…yes engage in activities and do them on a consistent basis, however, reduce the sports that will deplete you. Also, remember to allow full recovery after your sports.. Most people do not know how to do this properly. This is important if you want to regenerate and extend your life span.

It is important to structure your nutrition intake as to replenish and re-generate your body properly along with using the right supplements for muscle recovery. As shall be presented throughout this book, you will be given the keys on how to do this more efficiently as to maximize results.

Myth #2 Vaporized!

The Cholesterol Myth

In recent years the talk about cholesterol and how you need to limit to-tal levels every day for better health. Really? No thanks…just another funny myth my friend! Here is another erroneous theory that has no scien-tific basis whatsoever. Once again, people have done themselves a great disservice by following such myths. Pay attention because I keep things very simple.

Cholesterol is a required compound for optimum health. You need to ingest it in sufficient levels to maintain proper functioning of your body. It has numerous functions to keeping you young looking, vital and feeling healthy. The simple fact is, if you ingest the right kinds of fats then you will receive the healthy cholesterol type that benefits your health and longevity. If you do not ingest the right kind of fats then you are doing yourself a disservice.

The harmful cholesterol only comes from hydrogenated oils and fats that are chemically altered from their natural state. So, the key is to eat the right kinds of oils and fats and do it on a consistent basis. You won't have to ever worry about getting high cholesterol levels because your body will moderate it just fine because you are ingesting the right fats. If you ingest the wrong kinds of processed fats then that is when you will get high cholesterol levels.

So do yourself a favor, keep it simple and eat the right kinds of fats, very easy and simple to follow. Leave the rest, don't buy the hype and scam. There is no need to worry about high cholesterol levels if you eat a balanced and natural diet for your body type. **Another erroneous myth exposed and vaporized!**

The Eat Lean Meats Myth

In recent years there has been a shift of people starting to eat leaner cuts of meat such as chicken breast, lean red meat portions and other meats of leaner type. It is proposed that eating leaner meats is healthier than eating fattier portions of meat as in chicken wings and chicken legs and rib eye steaks and ground beef. Well my friend, yep you guessed it, just another erroneous myth being proposed as healthy. Let me simply provide basic holistic facts and common sense because that is all you require to see the Truth.

Eating lean cuts of meats actually promotes low levels of health and causes your body to become depleted of nutrients and creates an acidic environment internally. Lean meat is pure protein and requires extra enzymes and other bio-nutrients to break down the protein so that your body may make use of it to supply itself for nutrition.

Excessive consumption of lean meats causes all sorts of health disorders and places strain on the liver and colon. By the way, eating fatty portions of meat DOES NOT clog arteries as is being proposed. The clogged arteries come from other factors such as the consumption of unhealthy hydrogenated fats, excessive sugar intake which leads to yeast and parasite formation and other metabolic wastes in the body that accumulate. You may actually get artery clogging by ingesting excessive amounts of lean meats since the body becomes acidic. Then your body will have to take calcium from your system to buffer this acid. Thus after some time stones and deposits occur from the excessive free floating calcium.

Calcium is the main buffer mineral used by the body to neutralize acids and other harmful waste products. So in essence you are doing yourself a disservice by consuming lean portions of meats.

The Truth is that eating the fattier portions of meats as in chicken wings and legs and the inners of the chicken, rib eye steaks, ground beef (the fattier the better) and other fatty meats is absolutely healthy and promote good health.

The main thing is to moderate your portions. A portion the size of your hand is a great guide to follow when eating meats. Also be sure to balance your meal with enough fresh veggies. In fact, my recommendation is to always have half of your plate be fresh steamed veggies.

The main issue of today and why people are experiencing health disorders is that they have their portions and their meat options way off. They are eating big portions of lean meats, a large serving of starch food and a super small portion of vegetable. This ratio of nutrition causes acidity in the body which leads to numerous health disorders and places undue stress on your organs. The key is to alter the ratios and the meats options and then you are on the right track.

A healthy meal consists of a half plate of fresh steamed veggies or raw, a complex starch food as in brown rice, quinoa or wild rice, or whole grain sprouted bread and then a small portion of fatty meat as in chicken legs or rib eye steak. This meal is balanced and has the proper ratio of fats to starches to protein. Also, another fact to become aware of is that eating fattier portions of meats is actually easier on your body. Fatty meat is easier to digest and requires less enzymes and bio-nutrients to break down.

And...the secret that your body knows which is healthier...the lean or the fatty meat. This is so simple but again you have been programmed to go against what nature has intended. So, do yourself a simple experiment...or even just think about it in a common sense way...if you have 2 options before you, one is a plate of lean chicken breast and the other plate has 3 chicken wings...which does your body feel a pull toward? Which do you really want to eat? Which tastes better and feels better when you eat it? Pretty simple!

Your Body Is A Sacred Temple

Your body is a Sacred Temple and is the most amazing creation in the entire Universe. If you only knew just how many biological processes your body is performing each second, you would marvel in awe each day. And, if you knew just how intelligent your body is and how it is able to manage and keep order of the billions of biological functions it requires to simply keep you alive.

Your body is by far the most amazing creation in the entire Universe. You will not find another creation in all of the Universe that is so complex and awesome as your body and how it is able to do all that it does each day. Thousands of advanced computers could never come close to doing what the body does. In fact, your body is processing more information in each second than thousands of advanced computers.

So, the holistic science of your body is that it requires basic foundational bio-nutrients each day as to be able to use as fuel to perform the many biological functions it does. When the body receives these vital life giving bio-nutrients, then it is able to function optimally.

However, if you do not supply your body with these life giving bio-nutrients each day as is Divinely Intended to, then your body begins to function at reduced capacities and your ability to be healthy begins to be less. As such, the body begins to perform inefficiently and the homeostasis is off key.

When the body does not receive its foundational bio-nutrients on a consistent basis then you are setting yourself up for many health dis-functions due to your system not having the proper inputs to provide the necessary compounds to fuel your body. This is the case with many people in today's society. They are not inputting the proper nutrition on a consistent basis as to provide the body with its daily requirements. Thus, you get what you got with so many people being overweight and not healthy as they are not inputting viable holistic nutrition.

So, there are 2 main reasons why most people are not supplying their body with the proper inputs each day. One is that the food supply simply does not contain the hundreds of viable and life giving bio-nutrients that your body requires to function at peak capacity. What most people are unaware of is that a majority of the food supply is devoid of the hundreds of vital bio-nutrients that you require for optimal health.

This is due mainly because the modern agricultural practices have literally removed the healthy bio fauna in the form of living bacteria and fungi or what some call living probiotics.

These little bacteria are the True Creators of the hundreds of vital bio-nutrients that your body requires for optimum health. The modern agricultural practices are very unhealthy and have altered the soil ecology and as such you now have soils that are depleted and do not contain the living probiotics that are Divinely Designed to create the hundreds of life giving compounds for health and wellness for your body.

This is a BIG reason why so many people are not doing well these days. Most people are ingesting foods that are devoid of sound holistic nutrition. Your body can only go so long without its hundreds of life giving nutrient supply. The body eventually goes into survival mode and then begins to alter your hormone system. And by the way, hormones govern your metabolism which has the duty of converting food into usable foundational compounds that your body uses as fuel.

When your body goes into survival mode it begins to lower your metabolic rate and essentially begins to burn calories slower. This is a natural survival mechanism of your body. It is designed to keep you alive.

The issue with so many people today is that they are not supplying their body each day with the hundreds of vital bio-nutrients and the body has gone into survival mode.

As such, their hormone system is off key and then alters the metabolism to burn calories slower as the body thinks it is not being fed. Simply know that just because you ingest a food, does not mean that it is going to nourish your system. In the case with modern produce, most of it is deficient in nutrition so even though you may ingest it, this does mean you are nourishing your body. In fact, the way most people go at nutrition, is that they are actually depleting their body by ingesting nutrient devoid foods.

It takes energy and enzymes and other bio-nutrients to break food into usable compounds by your cells. If the food you ingest does not have the hundreds of vital bio-nutrients then you are using up valuable energy, enzymes and other foundational reserve nutrients of your body for no purpose other than digesting the devoid compounds. So, you are actually depleting your system by consistently ingesting nutrient devoid food.

Many people think that ingesting organic produce is a better choice for receiving more nutrition. Well, actually, organic produce also does not contain the hundreds of vital bio-nutrients that you require to be healthy. Again, it is the modern agricultural practices that have altered the soil ecology and the probiotics.

So, organic produce usually is not going to be the solution as many people think. What requires to be corrected is the soil ecology and the natural vital probiotics. Get the probiotics back into the soil and now you can supply your body with its requirements. The only issue with this is that it costs quite a bit of money to get the probiotics at optimal levels.

So, as you can see this is quite an issue that requires to be addressed soon because your body can only go so long without receiving its hundreds of foundational nutrient supply. At some point the body begins to break down and you set yourself up for many health dis-functions.

What I am presenting is simple holistic science. This is something you can easily observe and validate. So now you have one of the main reasons as to why so many people are unhealthy and overweight. The food supply simply does not contain what is supposed to be there and as such the human body cannot function at peak levels. This is why it is essential for you to learn how to structure your nutrition holistically as to increase your vital nutrient intake.

Another main reason why so many people are unhealthy and overweight is that many foods available in grocery stores are processed and contain toxic ingredients in them. Even so called health foods that you can find at health food stores are not what is being claimed. You require being more discerning about what you believe as companies are putting flashy labels on their products claiming "healthy" yet if you learn the holistic science of what ingredients they are inputting into their foods then you will discover something that is not healthy.

You must be aware that processed foods are not ideal nutrition for the body. They are altered from their Divine state and as such they can no longer feed and nourish your body properly. Here is a simple formula so that you can comprehend the simple holistic science of health and your body.

Your body is Divinely intended to be nourished via Mother Earth pure foods.

Foods from nature in their natural state are the ideal form of nutrition for your body. It is this simple. You cannot outdo nature by creating processed food compounds and expect to be healthy.

Simply look at life and society and there have many people who are depleted and malnourished. It does not matter if you fill your belly. The main point is your body requires viable nutrition in the form of Mother Earth foods. This is simple holistic science. When you go to the gas station to fill up your gas tank, you get the right octane gas, correct? You wouldn't input a compound like kerosene or diesel in there would you? That would totally mess up your car.

Yet, this is what a majority of people are doing each day through the food choices they make. They do not comprehend that it is not as simple as ingesting any food compound to satisfy your hunger. You require nourishing your body with the vital hundreds of bio-nutrients that are essential for health and wellness.

A majority of the food supply is altered from its Divine state and cannot sustain life for long. **Just so you know is that most of the food supply (even Organic) is now either GMO or hybridized forms of produce.** These altered forms of food cannot sustain human life for long. Your body simply cannot recognize the makeup due to the altering of the molecules of these food compounds. It is at the molecular level that your body breaks foods into and if you have a compound that is altered then your body will not recognize it as is Divinely intended to.

So, our society requires to wake up and learn the holistic science of health and then begin to restructure their nutrition intake as to supply the body with what is Divinely intended to feed and nourish it.

A byproduct of ingesting altered and processed foods is that it can cause the body to become toxic and depleted. For some it can actually cause weight gain as the body simply cannot process all of the toxic compounds from the foods they are ingesting. Your body requires many bio-nutrients to cleanse and detox your body of bio-wastes and other bio-toxins. If you are not supplying your body with its vital requirements then it simply cannot purge the toxic compounds out of your system.

As such, you have accumulations of these bio-wastes and bio-toxins and then the body will store them in various place around the body. In fact, your body must now protect your system from these toxic compounds and thus it produces fat globules around them to neutralize them so they cannot cause any harm to your vital organs.

This is what is going on with many people in society. Their bodies are extremely toxic and depleted and the body has accumulated many bio-wastes and other toxins and now they are overweight because the body does not have the energy, enzymes and other detox compounds to keep the body clean and slim. Thus, you have an overweight society that is also depleted of energy as their system is not receiving the vital bio-nutrients that create energy and vitality.

Are you beginning to see the dilemma of the health of society? It is not as simple as eating a little better and drinking more water. In fact, I will get into the water dilemma later. You must learn the holistic foundation that I am teaching, otherwise, you will be wasting time, money and energy. Most of the current health paradigms have no clue of these Truths I am presenting. They are teaching philosophies that are erroneous and in some cases counter health.

You must be careful as to what you believe especially with all of the health information out there. It is wild sea of information and most of it is not going to even come close to providing you the holistic foundation so you may be as healthy as possible.

As you can see by now there are a number of issues that require to be addressed otherwise more and more people will become overweight and unhealthy. The time has come for a Higher pathway for optimum health. This pathway is now here and I am presenting it in a manner that is simple and yet profound. The pathway I teach is based on holistic science and honors nature and your unique constitution of mind, body and spirit.

The Truth About Sugar

Sugar is by far the unhealthiest compound for the human body. It does so many negative things to your body. If you truly knew just how unhealthy sugar is to your entire physiology, you would never touch the stuff ever again. Let me present some basic holistic science perspectives on sugar and why it is the unhealthiest compound for your health and your evolution.

You see, sugar is a processed compound. At the fundamental level sugar cane is taken from nature, stripped of its healthy components and then you are left with an altered compound that is toxic to your system and can do so many other negative things to affect your health. Sugar stimulates your nervous system and impacts your brain chemistry negatively. It will actually make your brain become addicted to it and cause your brain to fire your neurons and neurotransmitters way too fast for health and wellness. Your neurotransmitters are there to relay information to many parts of the body for optimum functioning.

If you ingest sugar frequently, it will jack up your nervous system and then impact these transmitters to relay information too fast or imbalanced and thus you cannot have a calm physiology. Your brain body connection then gets thrown off and you have inefficient timing of information and relay of other vital communication between brain and body parts.

Ingesting sugar is also depleting to your system as it is not giving you energy as you think it may be. The energy you feel after ingesting sugar is your nervous system that has become stimulated and jacked up artificially. It is not pure energy and thus after some time, after the stimulation has worn off, your energy levels go way down. This is not healthy and is not the way nature intended for you and your health.

Sugar will also make your body acidic by lowering your body ph. If you comprehend anything about body ph, is that your body ph requires being within a specific range, otherwise, you set yourself up for many health disorders. Once your body ph has been lowered, there are now many factors that can cause you many health dis-functions.

Sugar also induces parasites and yeast in your body as many of these parasites thrive in an overly imbalanced internal body environment. You have many people nowadays who have yeast conditions and other parasitic causes and the link is usually sugar. As long as you are ingesting sugar in any of its processed forms, you set yourself up for parasites. As long as you have parasites in your system, you cannot be optimally healthy, not even close my friend.

Sugar is toxic to your system and can also put your body in survival mode. As such, your body will become toxic and thus it must protect your vital organ components. Thus, your body may actually produce fat globules around these toxins and now you set yourself up for weight gain. Sugar will also disrupt your liver function and metabolism because it will have a direct effect on your hormones.

Due to sugar being so toxic and stimulating to your system, it can cause your hormones to be thrown off key. Hormones govern your metabolism and thus you alter your metabolism by ingesting too much sugar or starchy food products.

Sweetened drinks are the worst compound to ingest as they profoundly alter your inner ph and physiology. This in turn can alter your hormones and eventually your metabolism. The drinks with corn syrup and other sweeteners in society that are so popular will cause you more weight gain and faster than anything else. My recommendation is stay away from all sweetened drinks, eve natural and organic juices and teas. These drinks are way too concentrated and can really mess up your hormones and physiology. It is not worth it.

Sodas are by far the worst sweetened drink as they have many negative factors as in they are loaded with sugar, they have phosphorous which is very acidic to your body and the carbonation is also a very acidic compound to your body. This makes this kind of drink a super unhealthy compound that has many negative implications to your health and well-being.

Sugar Impacts Your Evolution Negatively

Ingesting sugar can also stifle your Higher Faculties of Intuition and other Spiritual Abilities. Its impact on the brain is very unhealthy and causes the brain chemistry to be thrown way off. As I explained, your brain is functioning at a multi-dimensional level and processing Higher Dimensional information along with governing your entire body physiology. Ingesting sugar essentially does not allow your brain to connect to your Higher Faculties which you require to evolve yourself.

To evolve you require to be tapped into your Higher Faculties of Intuition and other Higher Faculties. With sugar in your diet, you are doing a great disservice to your body and also to your evolution. Here is the main reason: **Your cells and DNA are supposed to be vibrating faster than the speed of light.** Yes this is a fact! If you truly comprehend just how complex your body is and how many biological processes are occurring in each second then you will see that having your cells vibrating at the speed of light or lower is too slow for your body to function optimally.

You see, your cells require information in a steady stream of pulsing life force or what some call Chi. In essence, your entire physiology is running via energy in the form of information coming from your brain as a direct link from Universal Consciousness or Source. The speed at which this happens is way beyond the speed of light, in fact probably a multiple thereof. It has to be at this super-fast speed in order for your entire body cellular system to receive all of the vast quantity of information coming in.

Here is a secret for you: When the cells and DNA of the body vibrate slower than the speed of light, this is when health disorders begin to set in. The relay of vital information your cells require to function optimally is simply too slow for your major systems to keep everything flowing as is Divinely intended.

Picture your wireless internet connection and when things are ideal you have super-fast loading and processing and everything is good. However, what happens if your internet connection begins to get bogged down and your computer starts to slow up and you cannot even load websites or check email. You have had this happen before and it makes your internet experience not fun.

Well, this is what happens when your body, cells and DNA are vibrating below the speed of light. Your cells simply cannot function as they are supposed to as the relay of vital energy and information that each cells requires is way too slow for optimum functioning. Do you see this? I pray you do because maybe, just maybe, you will begin to change your perspective on your health and your body?

Ingesting sugar literally slows the vibration of your cells and DNA below the speed of light and thus sets you up for low level health.

By the way, your DNA is so much more than some base nucleotides as modern science says. Your DNA is multi-dimensional and is also processing information from Source. There are components to DNA that cannot been seen by human eyes or microscopes, however, if you truly comprehend what DNA really is and what it really is doing you would marvel. Your

DNA is actually like a multi-dimensional super Photon computer and is constantly changing.

How does it change you may ask? It changes as you change. It changes with every thought you have, with every mood you have, it changes with what is going on in your environment as in the space you live and where you work. Do you comprehend what this means?

My friend, your DNA is constantly changing based on the frequencies and energies you are supplying it with via your thoughts, emotions, nutrition, your home environment, your work place, your friends, the music you listen to, the tv programs you watch, the clothes you wear and even the people you live with.

Maybe this is the motivation you require to do a complete holistic lifestyle makeover? Until you understand life on this profound level as I am presenting to you then you will probably not make the changes in your life to experience shifts that will catapult your evolution.

This is why what I teach about holistic living is so profound, because it helps you to shift at the most profound levels and ensures you only input healthy frequencies and energies in, on and around your body as to help you to experience Higher levels of health and wellness. My friend, it is the only way for you to even begin to tap into your Higher Potentials.

In essence, your body and your level of health is a direct link to your evolution as a human being and for being able to tap into your Higher Potentials.

The healthier you are, the more you can tap into Higher Faculties and Higher Gifts and Talents as they will be able to come through since your cells and DNA are vibrating at faster than speed of light. Thus, Higher Dimensional information will be able to be processed by your brain and thus allow you to perform and do things that most people simply cannot do.

You will surprised to see just how much better you feel by simply removing all forms of processed sugar from your diet. In fact, within a few days you will feel a new sense of relief and calm and well-being.

There are many other food items that will have similar physiological effects on your body as sugar does. Most people are simply unaware that everything you ingest breaks down into smaller components. Many food items that people ingest actually will break down into sugar-like compounds.

Food items such as white flour products, white rice, cereal, potato chips, pretzels, corn chips, crackers and other dry brittle food items will get converted into sugar once in your body. As such, the physiological effect is that these food items can actually cause you to gain weight due to the effect on your metabolism and inefficient functioning of your entire biological system. These processed food items are not nutrition for your body and will only serve to lower your level of health. My recommendation is to stay away from these food items as there are far healthier alternatives.

I have written a recipe called **Fun Food Fantastic** that has some of the most knock your socks off meal creations. I have in the recipe book super delicious and healthy recipes that will satisfy your taste buds and be healthy for your body. You can go to Amazon.com or my website at

RinoSoriano.com

Part 3

The Secret Spirals of Youngevity

The Secret Spirals of Youngevity work as a spiral staircase that take you to Higher levels of health and consistently produce results. They uplift, energize, regenerate, rejuvenate, renew, revive, and create ongoing health, wellness and longevity because they honor and support the Divine inner intelligence of your body. You want to be on as many uplifting youngevity spirals as possible as to ensure you are continuously going Higher.

The spirals of degeneration take you to low level health and shorten your life span since they do not honor or support the Divine inner intelligence of your body. Most people are following daily habits that place them on these spirals of degeneration and thus experience low level health, shortened life spans and never really being able to experience life on a High level with happiness and joy in their hearts. The fact is that many health habits that people think are promoting good health are actually doing the opposite. I already exposed some of the erroneous myths that appear to be True, however, when you examine them just a bit closer they fall apart quite quickly as they do not validate themselves in real life.

So, remember, the key is to be on as many youngevity spirals staircases as possible in order for you to reprogram your body for youthfulness and longevity. The more consistent you follow and are on these uplifting youngevity spirals the more the results shall speak for themselves. Ideally, if you can embody all of the youngevity spirals you shall be in a unique league of people who experience life on a new level. You will also help change the current paradigm of poor health and degeneration to one of youthfulness and longevity by showing people what is possible. How cool is that my friend? **Happy Spiraling!**

Here are the secret spirals of youngevity that I know you have been waiting for. Please remember that even though some of these secrets may appear to be quite simplistic, they actually produce results that last. The key is in embodying them as a part of your lifestyle on a daily basis.

The 12 Secret Spirals of Youngevity

Renewal, Rejuvenation, Regeneration, Revival

The Holistic Pathway To Longevity

Youngevity Secret Spiral # 1

The Breath of Life

Your breath or as some cultures call it the Breath Of Life, is the most important aspects of health yet is never talked about in society as being a component for attaining and maintaining optimal health. How is something so simple and FREE so profound? Here are some facts for you: The breath is your access point to Creation, to Source, to Universal Life Force Energy. Do you comprehend what this means?

It means that your ability to breathe properly will have a profound effect on your health since it is your main connection to the Life Force Energy that sustains all life in the Universe. The Hawaiians call it Manna, the Asians call it Chi, the east Indian cultures call it Prana. Call it what you like... the main secret is that it is essential for life and more importantly for keeping you healthy.

Most people do not breathe correctly due to improper alignment of their spine, stress and other factors that limit or impair their full potential breathing. Thus, there is limited Life Force energy permeating the body which can lead to impairment of bodily functions. So, of all the secrets you learn here for optimizing your health potential, please do yourself a favor and embody this one first as it is FREE and so simple to do. Remember, it is the simple health habits that you embody on a daily basis that create a lasting effect on your health.

So, how do you breathe properly for maximizing your health potential? You may begin by simply noticing your breath going in and out. Then, start taking in deeper slower breaths and count to say 5 and then pause for 2 seconds and then release for a count of 5. There is no one magic way of breathing, the key is to begin breathing deeper and longer expanding your chest as to bring in more oxygen and Life Force Energy into your body. Simple, Free and has a profound effect on your health when done daily.

My recommendation is to take deep breaths throughout the day when you have some time to concentrate for just a few minutes. Begin by doing sets of 10 deep breaths and increase as you desire. You may also visualize as you breathe, taking in cosmic energy along with air and having this clean you out as you breathe in and on exhale breathe out all negative emotions, feelings, thoughts.

Youngevity Secret Spiral #2

Hydrate Your Body With Living Water

The second most important component to health involves drinking the right kind of water. You require the right amount of hydration every day as to ensure proper functioning of your body as to get nutrients into your cells and wastes and toxins out via elimination. What you may not know though is that simply drinking more water isn't going to necessarily benefit your health, especially for longevity. In fact, most of the water sources today are not the right kind of water that your body requires for health and longevity.

Your body requires a special kind of water for optimum health. In fact, this Sacred kind of water is the way nature intended for us to be hydrated. You simply require looking at nature and the Truth becomes quite apparent. You as a human being need water that is from a natural spring source as in a river or stream or some kind of running body of water. Pay attention because this is profound and can make huge differences in your life.

Water in nature is constantly flowing and spiraling (Universal Secret) as it travels down through rocks and mountains. What has been discovered for many years now is that water that flows in spirals as in rivers, streams, mountains and other such environments has a unique molecular structure that is ideal for human health and longevity.

Another important Truth of water is that it requires being alive and charged with life force. In fact, this is the most important component to water as this energy then gets transferred to you if you drink it. So, nature knows best and is the only True water source that your body needs for optimal health and longevity.

Nature is the only source that can provide this optimum source for hydration as water that spirals via rivers and streams picks up energy from the earth (earth is magnetically charged) and thus the water becomes charged with life giving frequencies.

Isn't it so beautiful that nature has the secret keys to optimum health? My main point is that nature has all the keys that you require for feeling and looking our best. How beautiful. If you begin to look at life with new eyes, you shall see a new reality open up to you. There is nothing mysterious about health and wellness. It is so simple that you miss it because you have been programmed to think otherwise.

When you have eyes to see, the Truth is right there looking at you. The question is where do you go to find this kind of water. As you are aware most water sources of today are polluted. Bottled water has become the normal source of hydration for most people. There are many bottled waters on the market today.

Well, suffice to say that most of these bottled waters are not in a structure that benefits your health in the long run. First, these waters are no longer charged with vital Life Force energy as many have been filtered to remove most of the unhealthy components. Filtering removes pollutants however it also removes healthy components to water as in the healthy natural Life Force.

Many companies are using reverse osmosis and/or distillation to process water to make it cleaner. There are also home units that you can use to filter water and make it cleaner for consumption. Well, again, even though you filter the water and make it cleaner does not mean that the water is going to be healthy for your body over long run. Actually, what is being discovered is that by consuming reverse osmosis and distilled water for a long time can impact your health in negative ways since these types of water are actually acidic.

Simply do a simple experiment by dipping litmus paper into the water and see for yourself how acidic the water is. In fact, most bottled waters will show up as acidic. The health benefits being proposed in favor of such water filtering as in reverse osmosis and distilled water are not True other than the fact that the water is cleaner.

When you process water (filter) in this way you actually strip the electrons surrounding the water molecules of their healthy charge and thus create a lifeless (no charge) water. You also change the natural molecular structure to the water and now create a water structure that cannot support your health over the long run. This lifeless water can't get into your cells as nature intended. This also means that minerals are not going to get to your cells as the natural molecular charge to properly charged water is essential to drive minerals and other bio-nutrients toward the cell from the nutrition you intake.

Another important component to properly structured water is that it helps to remove toxins and waste products out of your body. You need to continuously have toxins and pollutants being removed out of your body, otherwise, they accumulate and get stored in your tissues and organs which leads to improper functioning of your body.

So, you need the right kind of water on a consistent basis to experience a Higher level of health and also longevity. If you do the research, the cultures that experience great health and longevity do so because their source of water is from nature, is Earth charged and is unprocessed. It is quite simple yet you miss this simplicity because you are programmed to think otherwise.

Simplicity is where it is at my friend. Keep it simple. So, I know you want to know how do you get this water then if your only options are to drink bottled water or use a filtering system at your house, both of which are not healthy to consume in the long run.

There are a few ways that you can recreate a properly structured water supply. As far as our modern way of living, these are the only True cost effective and simple ways of recreating the molecular structure and charge to water to benefit your health. You need to be careful as there are many companies out there proposing that their water machine or product does this or that and has these health benefits.

Well, most of these interesting water products do not validate themselves. I have done the research and have a small list of products that I will recommend for better health and longevity. These validate themselves and are actually much more cost effective than some of these so called great water products.

I have discovered a few cost effective ways to do this. You may email me or visit my website to learn more about these products. They speak for themselves and are a much better option to what you are currently drinking. Please visit www.RinoSoriano.com

If you want to discover more about water and its True components then my recommendation is to get the book by Dr. Masaru Emoto, Water's Hidden Messages. This book shall knock you outside the galaxy for what he has shown with his experiments. Wait until you discover what water really is, mind blowing!

Before you begin doing anything else for better health, the foundation is to drink the right kind of water because it shall allow everything else to work better. **Happy Drinking!**

Youngevity Secret Spiral # 3

Cleanse Your Body Temple

Cleansing the body properly is one of the greatest experiences for you on your path to optimal health and wellness. The abundance of health benefits are profound and enduring. However, you require cleansing your body in the proper manner, otherwise, you are wasting resources. By engaging in a proper cleanse program, you will begin to eliminate compounds from your body that are impairing your health. The benefits are numerous as in healthier skin, brighter eyes, healthier libido, more energy, more vitality, healthier hair, and an overall sense of well-being.

There are many detox kits on the market today each one proposing that their products will do this and that. Some of these products may be healthy and semi-effective, however, what you must realize is that cleansing your body properly requires a number of processes and a bit of time. To do a 3 or 5 day detox kit is not going to remove years' worth of accumulated wastes, toxins, parasites and heavy metals regardless of what the kit says.

So how do you go about cleansing your body properly and cost effectively? I want you to be aware that it takes a bit of time to do so and with the proper tools and resources. Again, there are many products out there for cleansing your body, however, you require keeping it simple, otherwise, you will spend hundreds to thousands of dollars with little or no improvement. I show people a simplistic process for cleansing the body. Another important point is to cleanse in the right order and in the right sequence of using specific compounds.

For example, the best and most efficient manner to begin cleansing your body is to start with your main detox pathway which is your colon. You want to ensure that your colon is pretty clean before going on to detox your liver or kidneys or gall bladder. If your colon is sluggish or clogged then obviously it doesn't make sense to begin moving stuff out if you are already congested. It probably won't go anywhere anyway and it may contribute to lower health levels.

So, keep it simple and also you require using the right products that work and get results and keeping it cost effective. If you go on this on your own, you will not know what products to use, how and when and which really do what they are supposed to do. Just be aware that this process is to be done in the right manner for you, your lifestyle and your body type. The results shall speak for themselves.

One of the main secrets of cleansing the body properly is that by clearing toxins, parasites, and heavy metals from your body, you will automatically begin to increase your consciousness levels. You will begin feeling better on all levels of your being of mind, body and spirit. You will have greater ideas come to you, greater inspiration to want to go out in life and do awesome things. You see, toxins and heavy metals and even parasites disrupt your brain functioning never fully allowing you to experience your Higher faculties.

In fact, many of your moods may come from the impact of these toxins, heavy metals and even the parasites causing hormones and other biochemicals to be off and out of balance. These impact your brain functioning and thus may cause moods and other health related issues such as poor organ function. You may be surprised to find how happy you become as you begin to cleanse and detoxify yourself.

The key is to cleanse the body and then maintain this pure level of health. By doing so you will experience Higher levels of health, happiness and joy. Again, this is a simple process just of honoring your body and nature. Begin your cleanse program as soon as you can so that you may go out and rock this life!!!

You must comprehend that the proper hydration is the key to a clean and healthy body. It is also the foundation to detoxing your full system. Structured water is bio-electrically charged with life force and magnetically draws nutrients to your cell membranes. It also acts as a cleanser to magnetically bind to toxins and pull them out of your system via urine, sweat and your bowel. Structured water is the catalyst and the most important factor in cleansing your body properly.

Structured water also hydrates your brain properly. It provides the proper electro static balance so you brain can process the billions of synaptic relays. It assists in keeping your brain cool and provides magnetic charge to spark some of the neurological functions. Structured water improves your moods since your brain will have the necessary building compounds to produce the essential neuro-transmitters that create the feelings of joy and happiness. You can visit my website to purchase my LifeForce Elixirs that I have infused with life force energy and other vital compounds for turbo charging your detox efforts.

Youngevity Secret Spiral # 4

Quantum Nourishment

Nourishing your body properly involves more than simply eating foods and beverages. The key to really comprehend is that your body requires the proper ratios of nutrients and the proper hydration for you to experience supreme levels of health and wellness. Nourishing your body requires you intake the proper nutrition on a daily basis and knowing what supplements to use and when. This may take a little time to refine, however, my message to you is only you and your body know what serves you best as far as nutrition intake.

You require learning how to tap into your inner body intelligence and your intuition as to be your guide as to what nutrition is ideal for you. Also, remember that your health is fluid and changes over the months and so you require honoring this and go with what you feel inside adjusting your nutrition intake as you feel intuitively guided to do so.

I know this may sound a bit challenging, however, this is the only True way that you are ever going to fine tune a nutrition lifestyle that supports your unique body type, genetics, mental, emotional and spiritual makeup. Here is yet another super-secret that most people miss because they are programmed and are distracted from the Truth. So, the Truth is that your health involves more than what you eat and if you work out.

Your health actually involves your entire life and incorporates your full mind, body and spirit. Essentially, you have a unique body type, genetic makeup, mental, emotional and spiritual makeup, all of which determine what kind of nutrition lifestyle serves you best.

Also, your environment and home life also impact your health and need to be included if you really want to be absolutely healthy. Even your occupation impacts your health in various ways. So, it is time to realize that your health literally is impacted by your entire life and each decision you make requires consideration on how it will impact your health.

Where you live, who you live with, the colors in your home décor, the smell of your house, the clothes you wear and even how much sunlight coming in through your windows will on some level impact your health, be it good or not.

The Asian cultures have known about this Truth for quite some time, some will know it to be called Feng Shui. Again, call it what you like, the fact is that everything is impacting your health so it is wise to become conscious of this and makes decisions based on this knowledge especially if you want to feel and look well and live an extended life.

So how do you nourish the body properly? Well, what I have discovered in my experiences and through extensive research is that there is a common thread of Truth that applies to most people on the planet. If you take time to discover the nutrition intake of healthy cultures of today and of the past, the validation shows that the people that incorporate moderate to high levels of healthy fats and consume a varied diet of fresh veggies and fresh fruits along with small portions of select fatty meats and raw dairy seem to support good health.

Essentially, it is a nutrition lifestyle that incorporates fresh whole foods as in wild crafted vegetables and fruits, healthy oils, seeds, nuts, sprouted grains, naturally fermented foods and drinks and select portions of fatty meats and raw dairy. The select portions of meats are fattier portions derived from free range animals.

Also, there is use of sprouted whole grains in the natural balanced diet as this is a much healthier way of eating grains. The grains being used in the western world are not healthy and in fact quite degenerating to the system. Humans are not supposed to ingest large amounts of refined grains, especially wheat products that are first processed to remove the healthy bran and then have added synthetic nutrients to enrich them. It makes no sense whatsoever to process a whole food and then try to enrich and add back healthy components to that food.

The foods doing the most harm to people's health are the empty starches as in the white pastas, white breads, cakes, cookies, pastries, sodas of all kinds, sweetened drinks and other foods using bleached white flour. In addition to this, the use of processed sugar makes these foods a detriment to your health.

Sugar is one compound to completely leave out of your diet since it has so many toxic effects on your body. It is degenerating, stimulates your nervous system and impacts your brain neuro-transmitters. If you want to extend your life by many years then simply eliminate the use of white flour products and food items and beverages that contain processed sugar in any form.

You can easily tell which people who ingest processed sugars and people who eat natural, clean and whole foods with no sugar and white flour. Here's a secret for you: You cannot get cavities if you do not eat processed sugars. This should give you a new perspective of what sugar really does to your body. Sugar actually takes energy away from your body, even though you may believe it gives you energy.

Well, the Truth is that when you ingest processed sugar, the biological effect is that it stimulates your nervous system and is a false energy. In total, it will also strip nutrients from your body in the attempt to neutralize the toxic effect of the sugar composition. Naturals sugars from natural fruits provide pure energy because they supply the body with healthy sugar compounds and other vital nutrients in perfect balance. In essence, they give you pure energy. These are readily recognized by your body and the body assimilates these sugar compounds quite differently than processed sugars.

Also the empty starch foods and processed sugar products are the cause of why so many people are overweight. People simply don't comprehend how eating a plate of pasta or drinking a soda or other sweet drinks is going to cause weight gain. They have fallen for the myth that says fat and calories make you fat. Not True! What makes people fat is the ingestion of high amounts of empty carbohydrate foods and beverages that cause to the body to malfunction and become quite toxic.

The high carbohydrate consumption also causes all sorts of hormone irregularities and brain chemistry dis-function. Another factor is that by ingesting high quantities of starch foods and high sugar content foods and beverages, this stimulates the growth of parasites which bring in more health disorders and imbalances. These factors will also contribute to weight gain and other weight related issues.

So, most overweight people are eating the wrong kinds of food and are extremely toxic. They are also holding onto too much water. The water is external to the cells. This means that they are not absorbing water but instead storing it in their system. Since they are toxic, their body can not process this unstructured water through their kidneys.

They are also very deficient in key nutrients, in particular healthy fats. By simply adjusting these people's diet in the right proportions and drinking structured water, they shall begin to slim down quickly and easily, however, they also do require to cleanse their body since they are toxic.

By combining a proper nutrition lifestyle, intaking structured water along with proper cleansing of their body, these people shall finally become healthy and moderate their weight. Once again, so simple yet most people miss it because of all the erroneous myths out there that deceive you into thinking that this is some mystery. It is actually quite simple and it validates itself because life shall reveal the Truth to you.

So, if you want to feel and look healthier, then you require structuring your nutrition intake so that you ingest the right proportions of nutrients and a varied diet that fluctuates throughout the year based on available fruits and veggies. As I already revealed, a balanced and natural nutrition intake is a great nutrition lifestyle that suits most people.

So begin eating higher amounts of healthy veggies both steamed and some raw. Be aware that most vegetables require to be steamed out a bit. What you may not realize is that most vegetables contain natural toxins on their outer skins so they require to be broken down a bit and you do that by steaming on low heat. You want to intake vegetables for the fiber to assist in elimination. Vegetables are not healthy as claimed for nu-trients. They are mainly fiber and this fiber is an excellent cleanser to keep you regular.

The Asian cultures know of this fact and thus steam most of their vege-tables as to be a healthier form for your body. If you ingest high quantities of raw vegetables, you place strain on your organs and digestive system and your body will also have to deal with neutralizing the toxins. So, do yourself a favor and steam your veggies on low heat or roast them. This is a much better option for optimal health. Again, validate this for yourself. Embody this Truth and let it show you what is valid.

The Future of Food Is Here – Super Nutrient Power Foods

There is one topic that many people seem to be unaware of and that is the foods grown in the soils of today are quite deficient of key nutrients. This is due to over-farming and the use of inappropriate agriculture me-thods that actually deplete the soil and environment.

The main point to be aware of is that most farms in this country have low level nutrient soils due to the fact that the modern agricultural proces-ses have literally wiped out the healthy micro bacteria and fungi that are the creator of the hundreds of life giving bio-nutrients your body requires to be healthy. Without these living bacteria and fungi in the soil then the plants will simple not have the nutrients to sustain life.

For you this means that you are not nourishing your body for optimum health. So, what is the solution? Actually, there are 2 super awesome ways of getting foods that are super high nutrient content. In fact, the futu-re is to have foods that are super loaded with nutrients and where you require eating less to receive your daily nutrition requirements. The methods I am speaking to you about are growing foods hydroponically and aquaponically. In essence, this is the process whereby you grow vegetables in a liquid nutrient medium as opposed to using soil. These 2 processes are far superior to soil farming as they conserve resources, mainly water because they only use 10% at most of the water that soil farming does. The good news is that these methods of growing food are the most efficient way of ensuring you receive the proper levels of nutrients.

Also, the fact that these methods are quite simplistic to utilize and low cost to maintain compared to soil farming. Soil farming uses way too many resources to get a return whereas the hydroponically grown produce uses minimal resources and is super healthy for human consumption as the foods contain high levels of key nutrients. This translates into you being able to fully nourish your body for optimum health and longevity.

Your body requires key nutrients every day, so to ingest foods that are fully loaded with these nutrients are going to make a huge difference in your health levels. To maintain high nutrient consumption daily is a secret key for living a healthy and long life. I shall have more information on this topic on my website. **Happy Aquaponics!**

Super Health Foods For Youngevity

To recap, the following food groups are the healthiest forms of nutrition intake to ensure you receive adequate nutrient supply. Fresh heirloom veggies and fruits, Sprouted and fermented whole foods, fresh pressed oils as in olive oil, grapeseed oil, coconut oil, avocado and avocado oil, almond oil, walnut oil, palm oil and butter, homemade yogurt, fresh sprouted nuts of all kinds, free range raw dairy and select fatty meats.

In fact, butter is one of the healthiest compounds you can ingest. It contains natural sources of Vitamin A and Vitamin E and other healthy fats that make this a super awesome selection. You can even use butter as a supplement by ingesting a few small slivers in the morning before breakfast. Your hair and skin will love it. Try it and see!

Fresh fruits as in wild peaches, local cherries, pomegranate, persimmon, pears, kiwi, mango, papaya, star fruit, apples, blueberries, strawberries, raspberries. Goji berries are one of the most amazing fruits on the planet so be sure to purchase the best quality berries you can find. Eating goji berries on a consistent basis will do wonders to your health. Sea Buckthorn is also a life extending food and will do wonders for your skin and hair.

Gluten free breads are a great food to use for your nutrition. These contain complex carbohydrates, fiber and high protein and they are yummy. **Gluten-free oatmeal** is also a healthy option, just be sure to add some protein and coconut oil and spices as in cinnamon, nutmeg and a dash of sea salt. You may add sprouted nuts and fresh fruit to make a healthy homemade cereal.

For natural sweeteners, you may use the following: **yacon syrup, , pure raw honey, coconut crystals, banana puree. Stay away from Stevia...** the white stevia products at the market are not healthy, they are processed and are not True stevia. True stevia is green in nature therefore common sense shall reveal that a stevia product ought to be green as well.

Free ranges eggs, raw cheeses, goat yogurt, goat cheese, free range chicken (legs, wings, inners, thighs), free range beef (rib eye, 20% ground beef, ribs), lamb, turkey legs and wings, Alaskan Salmon.

Organic nuts are an excellent source of healthy fats and proteins. However, you require to soak nuts before ingesting them as they contain enzyme inhibitors on their skins. You do this by placing nuts into a glass bowl and covering them with water for 6 to 8 hours. This will ensure that most of the funny stuff comes out, you then simply discard the water and now you may eat them for a healthy snack.

Baked goods may be prepared using gluten-free flours as in **brown rice flour, sorghum flour, teff flour, quinoa flour, millet flour and oat flour, almond flour**. Gluten is a compound that is in most hybridized grains as in whole wheat, rye, barley and is not healthy to the human body. It may cause a number of disorders so it is wise to either limit or eliminate this ingredient from your diet. Essentially, grains need to be soaked and sprouted before consuming them, however in modern times this does not really happen for a number of reasons.

So, most wheat products out there are not healthy for human consumption for numerous reasons. One, they contain gluten which is not conducive to health, two they are not sprouted, three wheat tends to get moldy and is actually the main cause for why some people do not do well with these grain foods. Mold is one of the most toxic compounds on the planet. It can really do a number to your health so it is wise to eliminate foods that are made with hybridized wheat ingredients. Use the gluten-free grains as these are much better on your body and easier to digest. You may require to explore with the gluten free ingredients a bit, however, you will feel the difference. Happy Baking!

Time To Nourish Your Emotions, Mind and Spirit

You may have forgotten that you are a multi-dimensional being and have a mental, emotional and spiritual component to your nature. These aspects of your being require being honored and nourished along with your body. In fact, nourishing these aspects of your being will do more for your health than physical nourishment alone can. You as a human being have mental, emotional and spiritual needs. These aspects of your being cannot be seen, however, they have more of a pull on your health than physical factors do.

I think the time has come to become conscious of this fact and begin to honor and nourish these aspects of your health. As you do, you will experience Higher results in your health lifestyle. So, you can have emotional, mental and spiritual deficiencies that then lead to physical disorders and that contribute to low level health. Nourishing your emotions, mind and spirit is a process where you simply get in tune with your inner feelings and be honest with them.

Begin to have a closer relationship with yourself and deal with feelings and hurts from your past. Perhaps write a letter to express any feelings you have about a person or a place or an event that you know impacted you on an emotional, mental and spiritual level. Processing of these inner feelings is crucial for your health.

What has been discovered is that these inner feelings can impact your health and cause all sorts of life complications. The key is to begin to honor these inner feelings, let them express themselves and then transform them into a Higher energy form as in love and forgiveness. This will do wonders for your physical body and help you to feel more grounded and balanced. I recommend to have a coach walk you through a process that helps you to transform these inner feelings as it will free your energy to so that you may create Higher potentials with your life.

As you nourish your inner self with emotional, mental and spiritual love, you will see a new reality open up in your life and you will begin to feel connected and joyful. Your spiritual essence is who you really are and you simply require to remember and honor this aspect of your being. **Happy Quantum Nourishment**!

Youngevity Secret Spiral # 5

Energize Yourself

If you truly want to benefit your health and experience longevity then it is essential that you learn about energizing your body. Eating food is only one way to input energy into your body via nutrients and vital energy from most fruits. However, there are a few other manners in which inputting energy or Life Force into the body is more powerful and easier. One of the simplest and greatest ways to input energy into your system is to get grounded via Mother Earth. This means to connect with nature in some way, to touch your body to the Earth in some manner.

The easiest way is to literally go into your back yard and lay down in your grass for 15 to 30 minutes. This is actually one of the greatest health remedies and helps you to feel awesome quickly. So, if you have a back yard with grass then begin doing this simple practice 3 to 5 days a week and let the results speak for themselves.

Humans require to be connected to Earth because it supplies our bodies with vital Life Force and energies that recharge, revitalize, and renew our energies. Mother Earth is the greatest magnet and thus you need to honor this Truth and connect as frequently as possible. It is your lifeline to life so just do it. Again, very simple yet profound what you experience. Give it a try and see for yourself.

Going to the beach is also another great way to get connected and grounded. Why do you think so many people love being at the beach? It is because there are numerous elements in abundance there that serve your health well. First, there is the water element that is refreshing, cooling and healing. Then you have the sand which is literally fine crystals that emit life force energies. You also have the air element that brings in fresh oxygen and then also the sun which is the greatest source of energy.

Additionally, there is an abundance of negative ions in the air in beach environments that support awesome health by affecting your brain chemistry. It is quite beautiful that beach environments have all these elements coming together to serve your health. Again, I always say nature has the keys to your full potential health. So, if you can get to a beach then there you have one of the greatest ways to receive numerous health benefits all at once. **Happy Surfing!**

The key to energizing your body properly is to bring in numerous sources of energy on a consistent basis as to ensure you always have more than enough supply. Connecting with nature is the easiest and most cost effective and most powerful way to do this. Working out with weights is a physical manner in which to input energy into your system. By working out in the proper manner, your body creates many life enhancing bio-chemicals that help to regenerate and renew your health and give you lots of energy. Playing sports also brings in lots of great energy if you engage in the right activities and do them in the proper duration.

There are certain health modalities that also work to input more energy into your system. These include chi gong, tai chi and similar type energy modalities that help to flow energy in your body to be more harmonic and easy flowing for better health. These modalities work by bringing in more Life Force energy that is available in the Universe.

Life force energy is everywhere and you simply require learning how to bring this energy into your body to benefit your health. The results that you may experience are profound. Again, these require to be performed consistently as to receive maximum results.

The following is list of activities that also help to energize your system for better health and longevity. **Taking a bath, swimming, singing, playing musical instruments, walking in nature, sunbathing, making love with your partner, and simply resting.**

The following health modalities work to balance your energy meridians to allow better flow of energy throughout your body. Acupuncture, chiropractic adjustments, reflexology, tui na and massage therapy. These modalities allow your body to function better and support better energy flow which in turn supports better health

The Super Life Force Secrets

I am going to share some Life Force secrets with you right now that can significantly elevate your Life Force levels. So, this grand Universe is one Gigantic Life Force Power House. If you know how, you can pull Life Force from anywhere in the Universe. For example, you can pull Life Force from the Sun. You can do this by simply connecting to the sun and visualizing the sun rays filling your body with Light.

You can also connect to the ocean, trees and rocks. You simply connect and breathe in the life force. Always be sure to give thanks and be grateful for what you receive from nature. If you remember as I stated earlier that the Universe is ALL LIGHT and you can use this Light to illuminate your body and you can even use it to expand your finances. Oh yes you can!!!

You can visualize the Light and Life Force going into your bank account each day. Try it and see what happens. You will be amazed at what you discover. My friend, Light is the magic key to life, to your health, to your evolution and to your expansion. Begin embodying this wisdom and allow it to uplift you to Higher Potentials.

Youngevity Secret Spiral # 6

Rest, Renew, Revive, Rejuvenate

In order for you to experience optimum levels of health, you require to rest properly and allow for full recovery especially after sports or activities. Most people and athletes are not allowing for full recovery and replenishment of key vital nutrients thus the body goes into deficiencies by tapping into reserve bio-nutrients.

You also require the proper nutrition intake before, during and after sports or activities. It is essential that you learn how to intake the proper nutrition because you want to maintain your body in anabolic phase (muscle growth and regeneration) as long as possible just as a sprinter does for their sport and training.

An ideal way for you to intake optimum nutrition is to eat a balanced array of nutrients several hours before your sport. You then consume a high quality protein drink 30 minutes before your sport or activity. This shall supply your body with more than enough vital usable nutrients. During your sport or activity you want to consume structured water with electrolytes, trace elements and enzymes as to maintain proper hydration and also vital nutrient supply to ensure keeping your body in anabolic phase.

After your sport or activity you want to immediately intake a super nutritious snack or mini meal as to begin replenishing your nutrient supply and to help regenerate your muscles and tissues optimally.

You do this most efficiently by ingesting what I call a super smoothie composed of mainly raw nutrition.

Mystic Smoothie Recipe

1 Cup of Fruit as in Frozen Strawberries, Blueberries, Raspberries

½ Organic Banana

1 Ripe Avocado

2 BIG Scoops of Balanced and Sprouted Protein Powder

1 Cup Unsweetened Coconut Milk

This allows your body to receive pure raw nutrients as quickly as possible since the intention is to get nutrients to your muscles in rapid form. Most athletes and people who partake in activities do themselves a disservice by ingesting the wrong forms of nutrition as in processed sugar drinks or smoothies loaded with sugar and synthetic nutrients and low quality proteins. Ingesting high sugar drinks and snacks right after a workout or sport place your body in catabolic phase and basically limits the results you are attempting to achieve.

Also, to intake full heavy dense meals right after sports activities may take hours to digest and supply the body with nutrients. In this time, the body has gone into catabolic phase (weak, degenerating, deficient) levels. This manner of nutrition intake also limits and even reduces your results that you are seeking to achieve.

You may visit my website at **RinoSoriano.com** or go to Amazon.com to buy my book called **Mystic Smoothies, The 33 Most Delicious and Nutritious Smoothies To Rock The Planet**. These are the most yummy and unique smoothie creations that you have ever seen. Wait until you see the unique ingredient combinations and how delicious these are. These smoothies are like full meals loaded with vital nutrition that help with recovery and rejuvenation

Resting properly also applies to people who do not partake in sports or activities. It is important for everyone to allow proper rest and rejuvenation of their body. The human body is immaculate and is constantly working to keep you alive and healthy. There are times to simply rest and allow for complete recovery. This may take the form of simply sitting in your yard for the entire day and taking in fresh air and sun. It may also take the form of taking a bath and a back rub. It may take the form of eating wholesome forms of foods for the entire day. Or it may be literally sleeping the entire day and forgoing food altogether.

Listen to you your body, it is your best guide and it will tell you what it requires and when. Honor that inner feeling and knowing and you shall fare well. The body has its own Sacred Intelligence and so it knows what it requires and when. Learn to tap into this Intelligence because it is always guiding you for your Highest Good. Take a rest when guided to do so and the benefits will reveal themselves to you. Your body is your Sacred Temple, treat it as such! Happy Resting!

Youngevity Secret Spiral # 7

Live Your Passion

What I am about to share with you is going to give you a new apprecia-tion for your life and shall impact your health in beneficial ways. If you study people who have lived long lives you shall discover that these peop-le were living their passion and were active and involved in numerous so-cial functions. If you Truly desire to have the greatest impact on your life and health then it is essential that you be in alignment with living your passion. Living your passion entails being involved with activities that supply you with happiness, joy and excitement. Essentially they make your heart sing.

Living your passion literally gives you energy and promotes so many beneficial health enhancing qualities that I believe surpasses what nutriti-on can do for your health. Talk about energizing you and causing you to feel alive. The secret is that when you are in a joyful and happy demea-nor, your body is producing many bio-chemicals that are life regenerating and revitalizing. These compounds are a supreme quality of health pro-moting nutrients that create youngevity. So, discover your passion if you haven't already done so and then go out and do what you love as it shall help you to feel and look young.

Being in love has the same effect on your body as to maintain health and youngevity. By being more loving, you help yourself and the person you are sending love to. They benefit as their body then begins to create bio-chemicals that enhance their health and well-being. Check out Heart-Math Institute and what they have discovered.

This is why by being in Love is one of the greatest youngevity secrets to exist. You simply require learning how to maintain the feeling of love at a high level in order for you to experience the greatest results. Do yourself a favor, love yourself and love your partner and family members. You create a world of good when you do. **Happy Passion and Happy Loving!**

Youngevity Secret Spiral #8

Deprogram & Reprogram Yourself Now

Reprogramming your whole being is going to be the most important process you go through if you truly want to feel and look awesome and extend your life by many decades. You see, programming is very powerful yet is unconscious to most people. Programming entails all the beliefs and opinions you may have about a given topic. In the aspect of health, you have been programmed since childhood to accept certain beliefs and philosophies.

However, most of these beliefs and philosophies are not of Truth. They are lies and misinformation to purposely deceive you from the Truth. These lies are designed in such a way that on the surface level they appear to be quite true, however, once you begin to poke a bit at them, they fall pretty quickly.

As I have revealed throughout this book, many of the philosophies about health, nutrition and well-being do not validate themselves and in fact the Truth is usually the opposite of what is being presented.

You as a human being require to be more discerning if your Truly desire to be the healthiest possible. You do this by becoming more intuitive and sensing if something is of Truth or not. Your intuition is always with you and revealing clues if something is good for you or not. You will receive feelings about certain things and other times you will have a complete knowing that something is off or a lie. Begin using this faculty as it is your greatest tool for navigating the soup of life.

The fact is that most companies out there are trying to sell you something and they will supply bucket loads of so-called factual data. As great as the information they present sounds, it doesn't always signify that their product or service lives up to what they are claiming.

In fact, if you simply use your intuition and common sense, many times you can tell right away if something is just another erroneous myth. Most of the products out there do not validate themselves. So, be more discerning and learn to keep it simple. If something sounds too hyped up, well, there is a big clue that this product is probably not what it claims.

Programming works on subtle levels and is designed to bypass your conscious mind so that you simply accept what is being presented to you without attempting to validate or at least question what is being presented. Most of the information out there on tv, radio and magazines is loaded with misinformation that appears to be True, however, it is supplied in such a manner as to deceive you.

My motto is that if all of this information about health, nutrition and healthy lifestyle living were True, then I think by now millions of people would be radiantly healthy and happy and feel emotionally well. However, we as a society don't have that, do we? Not even close my friend, in fact, millions of people are not doing well at all and they have followed all the diet fads and other erroneous programs that simply do not support optimum health.

The Proof Is In The Puddin my friend. That is why I am providing my services to people, to help them remember simple Truth. To get back to nature because that is the only path to optimum health, always has been and always will be. Because of the programming though, many people have been deceived to think otherwise.

It is time for you to deprogram yourself now because it is vital to your health. Actually, this is the most important process to go through as it will allow everything else you do for your health to work as it is supposed to. Do yourself a favor, make the commitment right now, that you will begin to shed the erroneous myths and scams and erroneous beliefs that you have about the topic of health and nutrition.

You do this by simply going into your pool of beliefs and begin to look at each one you have, put it on the table and shine your light on it and discern if it is True or not. Chances are that most of the beliefs you have about health are erroneous so use this as a mind detox period to clean house. These beliefs are the main reason why you haven't been able to experience optimum health so why would you want to continue to carry them.

Visualize a big bonfire and throw them in because it will free your mind to take in Truth that shall serve you well and validate itself. You then go about reprogramming yourself by taking in new beliefs and opinions about health and well-being. You do this one day at a time and allow these new beliefs to become your new reality. I think by now I have supplied you many new concepts and Truths about health that will provide a solid foundation on which to build your new belief system about well-being. **Happy Reprogramming!**

Youngevity Secret # 9

Sexuality – The Super Secret of Youngevity

Your sexuality is the greatest aspect of your being. What many of the indigenous cultures have known is that your sexuality is directly linked to your state of health. Sexuality has little to do with sex per say but more to do with how you carry yourself and your energy. If you simply look at a person you can tell quickly how they are carrying their energy. Are they confident, are they shy, are they happy or are they sad? Simply observe and the Truth becomes apparent.

How a person carries themselves totally reflects what is going on within that person. This is related to their sexuality and how they feel about themselves deep inside. Most people are carrying low esteem beliefs about themselves and thus this reflects their outer demeanor and how they carry their energy.

You can easily tell the people who honor and love themselves as they carry themselves as they are beautiful and radiant. They usually have a sparkle about them and are magnetic. This is so because they are carrying their energy (sexuality) in a high esteem level. As within so without. As I have already mentioned the Truth is always present, you simply require the eyes to see. As you expand your consciousness, you shall have the eyes to see many Higher Truths that once you didn't see.

So, your sexuality has more to do with how you carry yourself and what you think and feel about yourself deep down. Yes, your sexuality is also about sex and love making, however, it is essentially how you choose to express yourself in any given activity. So, yes, how you make love to your partner is about sexuality, the question is... how do you express yourself there? Do you let loose and express yourself freely or do you limit your sexual expression? This will reveal many beliefs about yourself and how you choose to carry your energy.

So, begin to view your sexuality more in the light of how are you carrying yourself and your energy and how do you express what you feel deep inside. You can begin to change yourself quite easily by expressing yourself in a Higher way. You may choose to carry your energy as being more radiant, sexier, more magnetic, happier, more joyful, and more passionate about life. These feelings and ways of carrying yourself have a direct effect on your health and well-being. In fact, these feelings will nourish your body more than any food or supplement.

So, your sexuality is one of the greatest secrets for transforming your health and well-being and your whole life for that matter. It is your True essence so it is wise to become conscious of this fact and begin using this wisdom to improve your life. Become aware of how you carry your energy. Are you walking with a confident step or are you walking sluggishly and with low confidence? Are you walking with a happy glow or are you feeling down?

You can easily change these with a simple process of conscious intention. Walk As If is the expression. Walk as if you are confident and happy and successful. This is like taking off your shirt and replacing it with a super nice and new shirt that you love to wear. Imagine wearing this awesome shirt everywhere you go and now walk and carry those feelings with you. This is mainly an inside job. The outer always reflects the inner.

So, this is why some people are sexy and some are not. The sexy people carry themselves in a Higher way, they have greater feelings deep within about themselves and they walk knowing they are sexy and beautiful. Again, they are carrying their energy in a Higher expression. Everyone they come into contact with then feels this energy. This is why most sexy people are very attractive, it's the great energy they are pulsating out.

In the aspect of lovemaking it is essential to bring in this same confident expression. To allow yourself pleasure and to freely express yourself is vital to your optimum level of health and can extend your life by many years. Your human being-ness requires that you express yourself and the greatest way to do that is by connecting with another human being and making love in a natural way.

This means to allow yourself full expression through the act of making love. This has implications that can transform your whole life and catapult you to the Highest level possible as a human being. In fact, without full expression you are dulling your spirit and limiting your life experience.

Begin to allow yourself more free expression and carry your energy in a Higher way. The results shall speak for themselves. When two people merge in the act of making love there are so many regenerating and health promoting qualities present. I recommend studying Sexual Alchemy as these teachings reveal a much Higher way of making love and expressing yourself in order to increase your consciousness levels and to dramatically improve your well-being. Suffice to say that engaging in lovemaking on a regular basis shall help you to live healthier and extend your life by many decades if performed in a Sacred manner as the teachings in Sexual Alchemy reveal. View this link for a great book

Youngevity Secret # 10

The Fountain of Youth Is Already In Your Body

Ok my friend, are you ready to discover one of the greatest youngevity secrets to ever be revealed?

Most of the cells in your body replicate new young cells up to a certain point and then something happens. This has baffled scientists for years as human cells are programmed for health and longevity, however, at some point something seems to change or alter this. So what happens to cells to make them suddenly reproduce lower quality cells and degenerate? Well, there are many people attempting to discover what the Truth really is.

The answer is to look at DNA and genetics as there you shall discover what is really going on. Well, if you look at human DNA and use simple science, everything seems to operate via information or what is called programming. Just as a computer program is essentially a set of data (information) that is designed to perform a specific function or task, your genetics and DNA are also designed to perform specific functions.

So, essentially your cells and DNA contain programming (information) that instructs your body to be a certain way. So thus you get what the programming says. However, wait a second...because what I am about to reveal will literally knock you outside the galaxy. Are you ready to be knocked out of the galaxy? Are you sure? Ok...here is what I have been able to discover by putting pieces together. The programming (information) in your DNA and genes is NOT fixed as scientists say. The current paradigm says that your DNA and genes are fixed, meaning they cannot be changed. Really?

Ah, actually the Truth is that your DNA is fluid and changes every day. What does this mean? It means that your DNA changes as you change in consciousness. Every thought you have, every emotion you have, every belief you carry is all influencing your DNA and literally your health levels. Do you comprehend what this is saying? It reveals that you are creating your level of health and well-being on a moment by moment basis.

You can change your programming in your DNA by simply intending to do so and by thinking better thoughts, changing your belief systems and by feeling happier and more joyful. These emotions and new harmonic beliefs and attitude shall reprogram your cells and DNA to help you create a Higher level of health. This is why I teach what I do. To help you and others realize, hey, start cleaning things up because the sooner you do the sooner you get to experience better health and happier times. It is all connected my friend.

So my message for you is...do everything possible to create the Highest level of health because you then impact other people in your life and then they go out and impact others themselves and this is how we are going to change this planet. By everyone cleaning up their stuff and their bodies and their emotions and their whole lives and thus the whole planet begins to change. The results shall speak for themselves.

So, do you get it? You can begin right now changing the programming of your entire body by simply accepting new beliefs about your life and what you think is possible. You can also begin thinking better thoughts about yourself and feeling happier about who you are and what you have in life.

The paradigm that is currently out there is saying humans live to this or that number on average. Well, again, that is a program running in most humans' consciousness, so that is what they shall experience. Be careful of your beliefs because they are literally programs that have significant pull on your life. Stop believing the scams of life my friend. And this leads me to yet another erroneous myth to be exposed and vaporized right now. The myth that says humans live to this or that number. That is a lie and is not of Truth. It has been implanted into human consciousness over the years and now most humans live by that program.

We as a humanity can begin to change this funny program right now by beginning to discard these erroneous beliefs and reprogram ourselves for youngevity and optimum health. It is possible and it is the future and that future is RIGHT NOW! You can start right now by changing the funny programs that humans have allowed themselves to accept as Truth. The Truth is that you have the potential to live an extended life and experience a Higher way of living by being happier and more joyful and feeling more fulfilled. This is a choice you require to make within your own being.

If you do some research on indigenous cultures from around the planet and mainly from ancient cultures, you shall discover accounts of people who lived hundreds of years on this planet. They maintained great health and lived happy lives. How is this so? It is because they chose to believe and live in Higher ways. They lived pure lives and chose to create their own reality of what is possible for a human. Yes, they incorporated many healthy habits in their life by eating pure foods and drinking pure water, however, they also chose to be happy, joyful and believed on much Higher levels.

You have been programmed to accept certain beliefs about life and your health. Most of these beliefs are actually doing you a disservice. They are contributing to low level health and shortening your life span. Why would you choose to continue to carry these limiting beliefs. Begin cleansing yourself of all these funny beliefs and so-called factual data. Truth validates itself. It is a boat that floats. Most paradigms out there do not float once you attempt to validate them. In fact, they put you on a path of limitation and low level living. So, what do you choose? Happy Belief Vaporizing!!!

Youngevity Secret # 11

Sing From Your Heart

I believe singing or humming or toning is one of the greatest practices to incorporate into your daily life. By singing or toning, you help to create frequencies in your body that I believe help your cells to function better. These frequencies help you to be calmer and seem have a great effect on your body and cells. Singing literally raises your frequency and can elevate your mood. The next time you are feeling a bit down or emotional, simply begin by singing a harmonic song or start toning vowel sounds as in "O" or "E" or "A" or "U" as in AAAAAAAAAAAAAAAAAAAAAAA.

Do this for several minutes or for as long as you like. Explore with the different vowel sounds. Or you may sing from your heart as this is probably the best remedy for elevating your frequency and mood. There is something in your heart that you may want to say, so go for it…sing what you want to express. It shall do beautiful things for your health and well-being and it may even catapult your evolution spiritually. Give it whirl and see. **Happy Singing!**

Youngevity Secret # 12

Music Feeds Your Sprit

Music is one of the greatest blessings of life. Every culture to ever walk this planet has incorporated music into their lifestyle. In fact, some cultures use music in all aspects of their life as they feel it feeds your spirit. Well, again, this can be validated by simply observing and using it in your life. You know by now that music absolutely elevates your mood and at times totally pumps you up and at other times helps you to feel calmer.

The main point is that music has the ability to raise your frequency and promote many other health promoting qualities. I believe the greatest remedy for a person is to play a musical instrument as this expression allows for creativity and also to clear emotions.

Each musical instrument has its own powerful effect on your body so begin to explore with various musical instruments and see what it can do for your health and life. There are certain musical instruments that seem to have very profound effects on not only your body but also your consciousness. The didgeridoo seems to work on many levels of your being and can elevate your consciousness.

The secret is that the frequencies that travel out through the instrument come out in spiral formation. In most other instruments, the sound comes out in all directions at once or in waves. This is the main reason why I chose to call my book the Secret Spirals of Youngevity.

You see there is a Universal secret about spirals. If you simply observe life and the entire Universe, the Truth becomes quite apparent. **And this is…the secret that everything in the Universe is spiraling in some way…**there are tornados that spiral, hurricanes that spiral, and water that spirals.

Oh yeah, and the fact that DNA is also in spiral formation. Ah ha, another secret my friend. DNA spirals for a specific reason. It has to do with energy. The energy of the Universe is actually traveling in spiral formation. Thus energy flows in spirals whether in the Universe or on this planet or in your DNA. It is the most efficient way for energy to travel and to relay information. Most people tend to think that light travels in a straight line. Not so, it actually travels by bending and spiraling through space and beyond. As you can see, this spiraling movement of energy is a profound Universal Secret. All the indigenous cultures to ever walk this planet knew about this Universal Truth. This has profound implications on our health and our humanity as a whole.

In totality, energy is information and that information programs everything to do what it does. In the aspect of human DNA, the energy (information) within your body carries out specific functions. In the aspect of a tornado, the energy is simply carrying out the information that says to spiral or funnel and move. This entire grand Universe is literally one big gigantic stream of information pulsating out and carrying out unique expressions of life. In Truth, the whole Universe is programmed via DNA.

Each body in the Universe has its very own DNA signature. They are pulsating out a tune, a song if you will that is unique unto that body. So too is your body blipping out a tune based on your DNA signature and level of health.

If you have low level health then you will be pulsating out a weaker frequency. The stronger your health level then your frequency is much Higher. This is why you can sense a person who is healthy from quite a distance away. Their pulsating energy field is much stronger and goes out much further than someone who has low level health. This is why it is important for you to become aware that you can literally help change the people around you and this planet by simply creating a Higher level of health and wellness.

What you blip out affects everyone and everything on this planet. Just as a rock thrown into a pond ripples out to affect the whole body of water, so too do you pulsate out frequencies that ripple out and affect everything.

Are you beginning to see how important this is? Your level of health and level of consciousness can have a profound effect on this game called life. Everyone is important and matters and everyone is affecting everyone else. Do you get it? So, it is wise to ensure that everyone is as healthy as possible if we as a collective want to go anywhere. Having only a small percentage of humans on this planet be healthy is not ideal since on some level, the health of the others is going to serve to bring down the frequency of the healthy ones. It is all about frequency my friend. You ought to do everything you can to elevate your frequency for not only your sake but for the sake of everyone on this planet.

Your Higher frequency will serve to pull up the frequency of others around you. You thus can help to change numerous people in life by simply living a healthy lifestyle. You also serve as an example of what is possible for the others and show them the way through your lifestyle. Pretty cool stuff if you ask me. This only requires that you shift your consciousness level or your perspective to view this whole game of life as a pond and that what you do and pulsate out affects everyone else.

So with this Higher awareness you begin to live your life feeling connected to everything and everyone and see what the Indigenous cultures were and are attempting to tell everyone…and that is **We Are All One and All Connected**…what affects one affects the others. Begin elevating your frequency and see what beauty becomes visible in your life. **Happy Pulsating!**

The Youngevity Revolution

Are You Game?

Well, I think I have given you more than enough to contemplate for now and a foundation that shall serve you to improve your entire life if you allow it. I have revealed the greatest health wisdom and knowledge for helping you to live a happier, healthier and a super long life. It is time for you to embody what you have learned. Start with one life principle and make it a part of your daily life before bringing in another.

This way within 3 months' time you shall have incorporated most if not all of the secret spirals of youngevity. This shall place you in a unique league of people who get to experience life on a much Higher level. From this Higher level you shall create more beauty and be able to help others in a more efficient way as being an example of what is possible.

I now offer you a mission of monumental proportions. My mission to you is do everything possible to create the greatest level of health for your life. Invest in cleaning your body out and learning how to structure the proper nutrition lifestyle for your body type and unique makeup. Listen, when you feel and look fantastic you want to go out and do amazing things. When you feel so good that you just want to go out and play and make other people happy. This state of being is possible for you and is actually your True nature.

We are all supposed to feel and look young, healthy, and happy. However, in this modern society, it has become a challenge to be absolutely healthy and happy. Way too many distractions and low quality food preparations and the forgetting of simple Truth for health and wellness.

Get back on track because as you do then your life improves and then you provide an example for others to do the same. Clean yourself and your whole lifestyle up and see what happens. It is actually so simple yet you have missed because of all the distractions and illusions that have been presented to you. Get grounded right now and begin to embody the spirals of youngevity in your life. I am here to help you in any way I can. I am willing to provide you the proper coaching and guidance to get you feeling and looking your absolute best. This is to be done not only for you but for the entire planet.

As you clean up and harmonize your lifestyle, people in your life and environment will want what you got. They will come to you for guidance and ask you how you did it. In sharing your Truth, you allow other people to awaken to their Truth. Look my friend, creating optimum health is the wave of the future and that future is now. It is all going there anyway so why not join in the fun today and begin your path and journey to optimum health and youngevity.

More and more people are waking up and cleaning themselves up to live healthier and happier lives. It is the only way we as a collective humanity are going to shift this disharmonic reality to one of beauty and harmony. You have an impact on this game and you have the ability to impact people in your life beginning today by the choices you make. By choosing to create optimum health, you set in motion a wave that impacts many others in ways you shall not comprehend. However, you will eventually see the results as people in your life begin to change their lifestyle. Join the revolution my friend.

It is going there anyway so why not join in the fun and have a big hand in the creation of a new reality... a reality where most people are vibrantly healthy and creating beauty with their lives. This reality benefits everyone on the planet as people who are radiantly healthy also have a Higher level of consciousness and with this consciousness create beauty that benefits all. You can be one of these people within a few months from now if you begin right now to clean up and embody Higher living principles and habits for health and youngevity. The foundation has been set, it is now time for you to walk the path, a path to your Higher Potential.

I wish you many blessings on your journey to youngevity.

To Your Health,

Rino Soriano - The Health Alchemist

Rino Soriano's Bio

Holistic Health Intuitive, Clairvoyant Life Coach, Spiritual Author, Spiritual Luminary. Utilizing his spiritual gifts of heightened clairvoyance and intuition, Rino Soriano is a Dynamic Life Force who guides his clients to access their inner power and activate their Life Force.

As a spiritual intuitive and clairvoyant, Rino is able to tune in and see Higher Possibilities that you may not have considered in your life. His specialty is aligning your Life Force and optimizing your nutrition intake to match your level of Being so that your Higher Faculties can kick in and provide the catalyst you require for your evolution. Rino's guidance and mentoring will accelerate your evolution with spiritual insights and practices that get results.

Rino also speaks on the topic of Consciousness and shall uplift your perspective of just how valuable you truly are and how important you are in the evolution of the planet. Through his luminary perspectives and revolutionary holistic practices, Rino is guiding beings of Higher Consciousness to assist them in accessing their Higher Faculties as to use for The Greater Good Of All. Rino's expansive perspective about life and humanity's Higher Potential entails leaving a legacy for future generations to marvel at.

If you want to discover more about Rino and how he helps people to experience youngevity, please visit:

www.RinoSoriano.com Rino has monthly coaching programs where he walks you step by step toward creating youngevity and tapping into your full potential.

You can also visit his website to view his holistic web store with High Frequency products and resources in helping you to experience youngevity.

You can go to Amazon.com to view or purchase Rino's other books.

Body Brilliance, The 8 Royal Diamonds For A Healthier and More Radiant You

Sensational Slimming Secrets, A Revolutionary Pathway To A Healthier and Slimmer You

Fun Food Fantastic, Knock Your Socks Off Meal Creations

Mystic Smoothies, The 33 Most Nutritious and Delicious Smoothies To Rock The Planet

Consciousity, The Crystalline Key For Transforming Earth Blue

Bodybuilding Brilliance, Massive Muscle Makeover

Sports Brilliance, A Holistic Pathway For Your Higher Sports Performance

Produced by Flying Hawk Productions™